Visit
CALIFORNIA
Farms

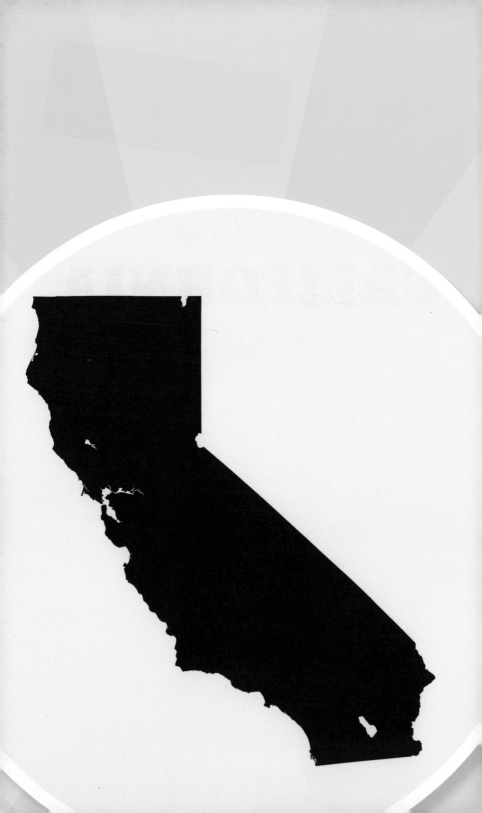

Visit CALIFORNIA *Farms*

YOUR GUIDE TO FARM STAYS, TOURS, AND HANDS-ON WORKSHOPS

ERIN MAHONEY HARRIS

 WILDERNESS PRESS . . . *on the trail since 1967*

Visit California Farms: Your Guide to Farm Stays, Tours, and Hands-On Workshops

First edition, first printing

Copyright © 2016 by Erin Mahoney Harris

Project editor: Ritchey Halphen
Cover and interior photos © 2016 by Erin Mahoney Harris, except where noted
Cover design: Scott McGrew
Book design: Jonathan Norberg
Cartography: Steve Jones
Copyeditor: Kate McWhorter Johnson
Proofreader: Rebecca Henderson
Indexer: Sylvia Coates

Cataloging-in-Publication Data is on file with the Library of Congress.

ISBN: 978-0-89997-789-8; eISBN: 978-0-89997-790-4

Manufactured in the United States of America

Distributed by Publishers Group West

WILDERNESS PRESS
An imprint of AdventureKEEN
2204 First Ave. S., Suite 102
Birmingham, AL 35233

Visit wildernesspress.com for a complete listing of our books and for ordering information. Contact us at info@wildernesspress.com, facebook.com/wildernesspress1967, or twitter.com/wilderness1967 with questions or comments.

Cover photos: (Front cover, clockwise from top) California Citrus State Historic Park, Hidden Villa, Full House Farm, The Farm in Salinas, Earthworks Farm, Toluma Farms. (Back cover, top to bottom) Fairview Gardens, Green String Farm

DEDICATION

This book is dedicated to Tony and to our children, West and Avery, my frequent travel companions and my most compelling reasons for caring so deeply about a sustainable future for our food supply and our planet.

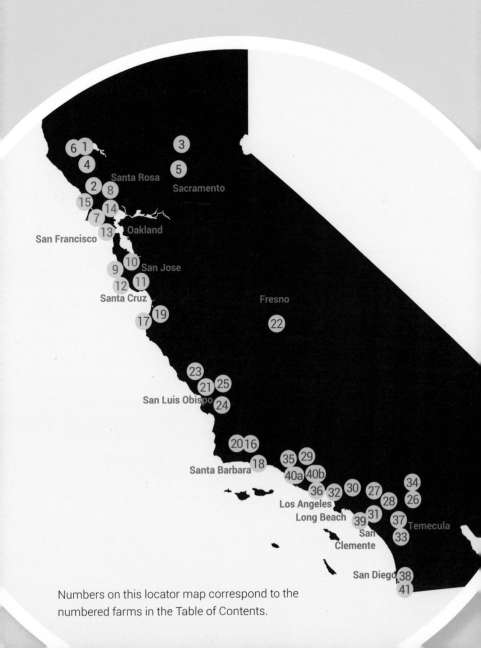

Numbers on this locator map correspond to the numbered farms in the Table of Contents.

TABLE OF CONTENTS

ADDITIONAL FARMS IN THE AREA

A Brief Glossary of Sustainable-Farming Terminology

Index

About the Author

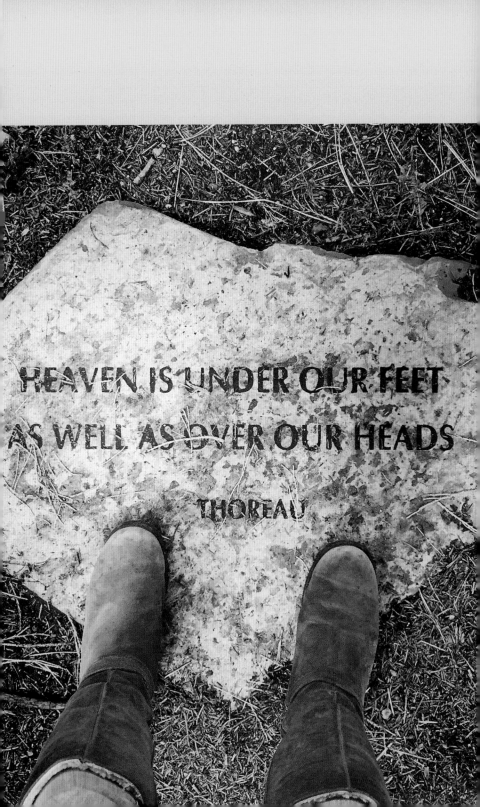

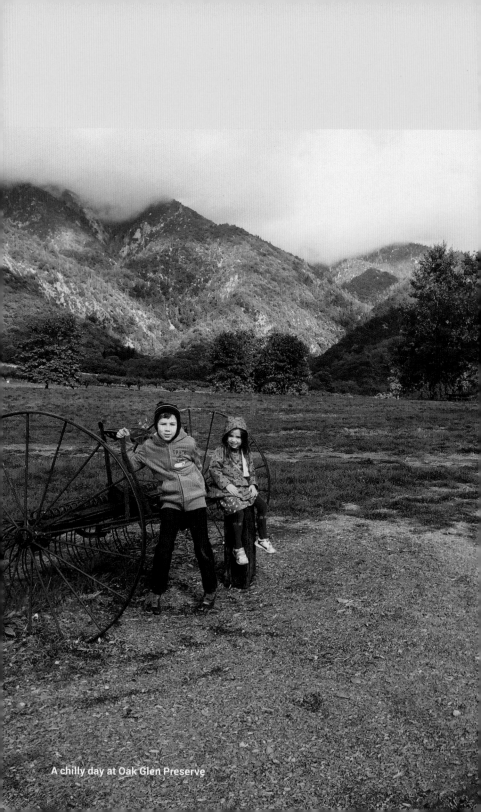

A chilly day at Oak Glen Preserve

INTRODUCTION

WITH ITS YEAR-ROUND SUNSHINE, beautiful and varied topography, and relatively mild climate, California has historically been an agricultural Shangri-la, encompassing all manner of farms, orchards, vineyards, and ranches. But the Golden State has struggled with a devastating drought in recent years, lending even more urgency to the growing sustainable-farming movement.

This guide spotlights the smaller-scale, family-owned farms, vineyards, and ranches that have expanded their operations beyond agriculture into hospitality and education, opening their doors to visitors to offer a deeper look at rural life and how to produce food sustainably and responsibly. It's written for everyone who cares about where our food comes from and how agriculture affects the planet, whether you're a parent yearning to teach your children valuable life skills, an outdoors enthusiast, an environmentalist, an avid gardener, an adventurous foodie, or simply someone looking for a new and enlightening travel experience.

Visiting the farms featured here will take you to some of the most gorgeous parts of the state, from breathtaking coastal cliffs to oak-studded foothills to rolling orchards and vineyards. And while I positively basked in all of the natural and pastoral beauty during my travels, by far the most rewarding part of writing this book was getting the chance to know so many farmers. Observing firsthand—and sometimes participating in—the immense amount of preparation, planning, labor, and sacrifice that goes into running a farm gave me even more respect for the men and women who devote their lives to producing food for other people. When you do go on a farm stay, tour, or visit, I encourage you to spend some time chatting up your hosts; I guarantee that you'll be blown away by their breadth and depth of knowledge. As a nonfarmer, I would never be so audacious as to claim I know a lot about farming. What I can say with confidence after my experience researching this book is that I have *learned* a LOT about farming.

My hope is that this guide will in turn give you a better understanding of how our food is produced, along with the skill, dedication, patience, and hard work required to produce it responsibly. With any luck, you may even be inspired by your travels to start farming yourself, whether that means a few containers on the patio, a backyard chicken coop, a community or school garden, or even an honest-to-goodness ranch in the country. Because one thing is certain: The world needs more passionate and sustainable farmers.

—*Erin Mahoney Harris*

AUTHOR'S NOTE

CALIFORNIA IS A BIG STATE. It's also the nation's top agricultural producer. This adds up, as you can imagine, to a huge number of farms. And even though only a fraction of those farms are open to the public, agritourism, urban farming, and agricultural education are all—thankfully—on the rise, both in the Golden State and throughout the country.

In this book, I have spotlighted 41 farms, all of which I've been fortunate enough to visit in person. But as much as I would've loved it, I couldn't make it to every single farm in the state that offers public programs, tours, and/or lodging during the year and a half I spent doing my research. For this reason, I've also included a list of additional farms in each chapter that I believe to be worth checking out. As you use this book to plan your excursions, be sure to consult these lists to see what other agricultural tours, events, and farm stays are available in the area you're visiting. Keep in mind that the programs offered vary by season and, despite California's mild climate, some farms close for the winter, so it's always wise to call ahead before dropping by.

Although I have written this book to be as comprehensive an agri-tourism guide as possible, an enthusiastic and adventurous traveler is bound to make new discoveries. In my experience, the best way to find out about more farms and attractions in any given area is by talking to the farmers you meet, the restaurant owners who source from local growers, and even your fellow patrons at neighborhood coffee shops and cafés. Most farms are located in or near small towns, and most farmers don't have a whole lot of free time to devote to marketing, public relations, and website development, so you're most likely to discover a region's hidden gems by talking to the locals.

CALIFORNIA FARMS BY THE NUMBERS

10 GREAT FARM VISITS FOR KIDS

10 FARMS WITH COMFORTABLE OVERNIGHT ACCOMMODATIONS

● Northern California   ● Central California
● San Francisco Bay Area   ● Southern California

5 LOVELY FARMS FOR A ROMANTIC WEEKEND

10 FARMS WHERE YOU CAN GET YOUR HANDS DIRTY

5 FARMS THAT SERVE DELICIOUS FOOD

5 FARMS WITH HIGHLY EDUCATIONAL TOURS

Northern
CALIFORNIA

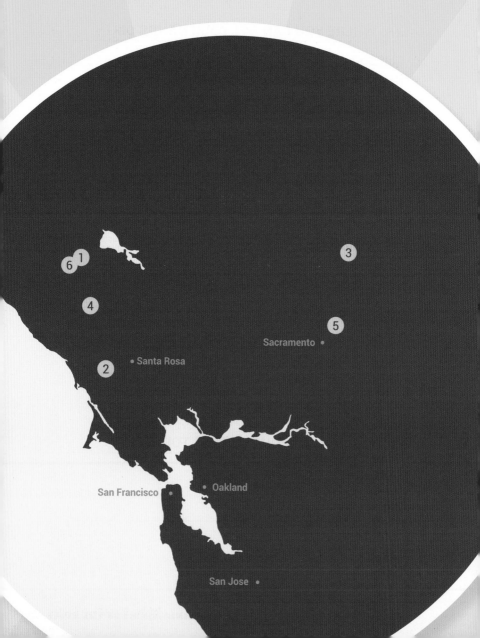

Sacramento

Santa Rosa

San Francisco • Oakland

San Jose

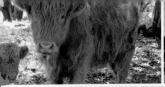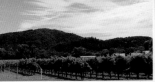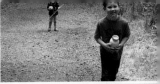

FARMS TO VISIT IN NORTHERN CALIFORNIA

1 CAMPOVIDA

13601 Old River Road, Hopland, CA 95449; 707-400-6300, campovida.com; open year-round. Detailed driving directions: campovida.com/hopland-the-farm

WHAT THEY OFFER Event venue, tasting, tours

AS YOU HEAD NORTH ON HIGHWAY 101, you know you're about to cross into Mendocino County when the road gains in elevation and becomes curvy and the meandering vineyards give way to craggy rocks and oak-covered hillsides. An official roadside sign provides confirmation with the slogan EXPERIENCE MENDOCINO COUNTY: WILDERNESS, WAVES, WINERIES. The unofficial fourth "W"—weed—doesn't appear on the sign, but it may as well; Mendocino County is widely known to be "green" in more than one sense of the word. But this book isn't about those kinds of farms, so today the focus is on Campovida in Hopland.

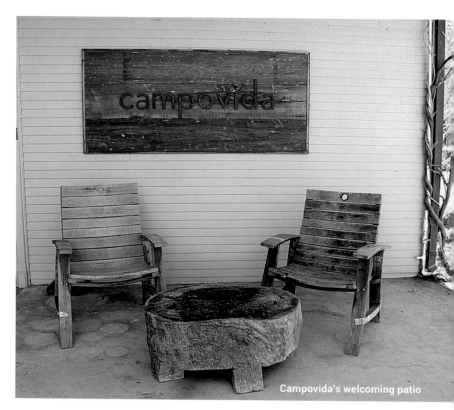

Campovida's welcoming patio

Despite its location off the beaten path in a tiny rural town, Campovida feels as refined as any Napa Valley winery. The property dates back to the 1890s, but the buildings have all been refurbished and redesigned. The land, meanwhile, has gone through several transformations over the years. It has a history as a hops farm (this is Hopland, after all), a stud ranch, and a Fetzer winery, and it even belonged to the liquor company that owns Jack Daniel's for a short time. During its tenure, the Fetzer family established a learning garden on the premises in the 1980s, which continues to thrive today.

The current owners, Gary Breen and Anna Beuselinck, bought the property in 2010 and, acknowledging that it won't belong to them forever, consider themselves stewards of the land, tasked with maintaining its integrity far into the future. To that end, Campovida, like many Mendocino wineries, is certified organic. Production is relatively modest—3,000 cases a year, which is much less than the land is capable of producing—but the emphasis here isn't on maximum productivity or profits. The owners make it their mission to honor the region, the grapes, and the ground, rather than producing the greatest number of varietals.

Until fairly recently, many of Mendocino's grape farmers shipped their harvest to winemakers in the more well-known regions of Napa Valley and Sonoma County. But more and more local farmers have become winemakers in recent years, which makes Mendocino kind of the Wild West of wine regions. The topography here is well suited to growing wine grapes; from hot inland areas to protected valleys to cool coast, the incredible diversity of microclimates and temperature fluctuations makes this an especially dynamic grape-growing region. Campovida grows its own Viognier and Sangiovese varietals and works with other regional growers to produce a wide range of other varietals as well.

Part of what sets Campovida apart from other wineries is its expansive learning garden and commitment to biodiversity. An olive orchard (Campovida also makes its own olive oil), the hundreds of varieties of plants that grow on the property, and eight beehives serve to break up the monoculture of growing grapes, contributing to both a healthier crop and a more resilient piece of land. The tasting room staff will happily provide you with a map of the property, encouraging you to explore the 6-acre garden. If you're lucky enough to visit the garden in solitude, you may find yourself in a blissful reverie as you wander its paths, enjoying the sights and scents of flowers, vegetables, herbs, and fruit trees accented with whimsical wood and metal sculptures. Beyond the garden are free-ranging chickens and beehives, creating a fully self-sustaining ecosystem in the most picturesque fashion. Guided garden tours are also sometimes offered at Campovida; peruse the Upcoming Events section on the website to find out when these are available.

Of course, a visit to Campovida wouldn't be complete without tasting what it has to offer. Wine and olive oil samplings are offered at Taste of Place, a.k.a. the tasting room. There is also a 10-room lodging facility on the premises, but the rooms are available exclusively to Campovida's wine club members and to those who host a special event on the property. If you're looking for other places to stay in the area, sister property Piazza de Campovida (see below) features an inn, as well as a pizzeria and beer tavern.

NEARBY ATTRACTION AND LODGING Piazza de Campovida

If you're looking for luxurious lodging, a tasty bite, or a cold beer in the Russian River Valley, Piazza de Campovida has you covered on all three counts. The inn offers deluxe suites for weary travelers, and the pizzeria serves delicious Neapolitan-style pies that pair perfectly with the custom-brewed beers from Linden Street Brewery, which are also served in the taverna.

13441 S. US 101, Hopland, CA 95449; 707-744-1977, piazzadecampovida.com

2 FULL HOUSE FARM

1000 Sexton Road, Sebastopol, CA 95472; 707-829-1561, fullhousefarm.com; open year-round

WHAT THEY OFFER Classes and workshops, lodging, U-pick

A STAY AT FULL HOUSE FARM, in the ultra-laid-back town of Sebastopol in the Sonoma Valley, can be tailored to suit just about anyone's preferences. If you're eager to get your hands dirty with some real farming experience, Full House has you covered—you'll be invited to interact with the animals and harvest your own dinner. But if you're more in the mood for sipping a glass of local wine in a hot tub and simply reveling in the impossibly beautiful pastoral setting, you can do that too.

Several lodging options are available on the property. The 2,000-square-foot guesthouse is ideal for a large family; with three bedrooms and several convertible couches, it can sleep up to 12 guests. It also boasts all the comforts of home (and then some) with a fully equipped kitchen, high-speed Internet, streaming movies and music, a DVD player and movie collection, video games, board games, and the aforementioned

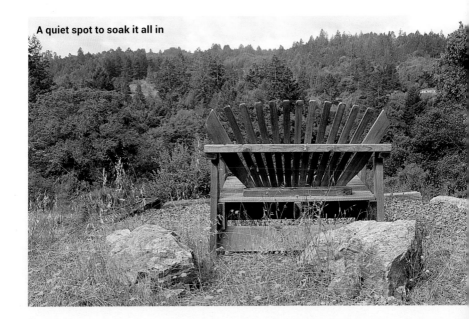

A quiet spot to soak it all in

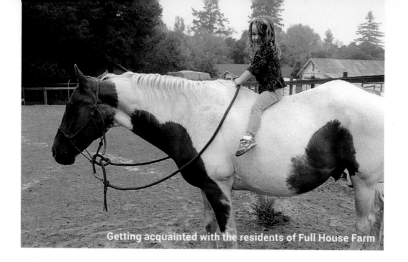
Getting acquainted with the residents of Full House Farm

outdoor hot tub. The home's great room and dining area have floor-to-ceiling windows looking out on redwood-covered hillsides, and you also have the option of eating outside on the peaceful patio.

Full House can comfortably accommodate small groups, couples, and individual guests, as well. A small studio cottage also has a fully equipped kitchen and suits one to two guests with a pillow-top queen bed set beneath a skylight. It too has a TV, DVD player, video collection, and board games, as well as a two-person hot tub out on the private deck. The final option is the fully equipped, self-contained farm-stay trailer, which also has a private deck with its own hot tub. All three vacation rentals are located at the top of the property, affording spectacular views of the surrounding woodlands.

Next to the main guesthouse is a huge garden with fruits and veggies for the picking. Your host will greet you upon arrival and give a brief tour of what's ready to be harvested. From there on out, you're free to pick and gather to your heart's content for the duration of your stay. All guests will find their kitchen stocked with freshly gathered eggs from the henhouse, a fresh loaf of bread from Wild Flour Bread down the road (see sidebar), and a bottle of local Sonoma County wine. You can supplement these provisions with additional farm-raised delicacies such as fresh goat's milk, kefir, yogurt, and cheese. These items are available for purchase on the honor system in a refrigerated box next to the farmhouse, which is a short walk down the hill from the guesthouse.

Full House Farm offers tours free to all farm-stay guests and for a small fee to day visitors. Farm proprietor Christine Cole or one of the assistants who reside on the farm will walk you through a 90-minute to 2-hour lesson on how truly sustainable, humane, small-scale farming works. You'll have the opportunity to feed the goats, gather eggs from the chickens, and even shovel horse manure if you're up for it. At the end of the tour, you're treated to a tasting of the farm's incredibly fresh-tasting goat's milk, cheeses, and homemade preserves. In season, apple and pear picking are also on offer at Full House Farm.

NEARBY ATTRACTION Wild Flour Bread

Wild Flour Bread is in a tiny village in Freestone Valley, between Sebastopol and Bodega Bay on the appropriately named Bohemian Highway. The brick-oven bakery is tended by a group of friendly young folks with glowing complexions who are happy to let you sample their assortment of creative baked goods, such as sweet loaves studded with pears, figs, and candied ginger; herbed goat cheese flatbread; and dark chocolate hazelnut biscotti.

Wild Flour's products are available for sale only in the bakery because, as they say, they want to meet and get to know their customers. They don't offer it wholesale, which is all the more reason to stop by and pick up a couple of loaves if you're in this neck of the woods on a Friday, Saturday, Sunday, or Monday.

But despite the bakery's commitment to community and exceptional baked goods, the best thing about it may be the bountiful garden. The plot has been whimsically and lovingly cultivated with pea and green bean tunnels, abundant flowering vines, and towering sunflowers, along with just about any other fruit or veggie you'd want to find growing in a well-stocked kitchen garden. Guests to the bakery are free to explore but gently asked not to pick and plunder.

140 Bohemian Highway, Freestone, CA 95472; 707-874-2938, wildflourbread.com

3 LONG DREAM FARM

Lincoln, CA; 916-543-0758, longdreamfarm.com; open year-round. Call, e-mail farminfo@longdreamfarm.com, or use the website contact form to obtain directions or book a tour or stay.

WHAT THEY OFFER Lodging, tours

CONSIDER YOURSELF WARNED: A trip to Long Dream Farm may make you entirely rethink the way you've chosen to live your life, particularly if you're a city dweller. In other words, this Animal Welfare Approved family farm represents agricultural life at its most idyllic. That isn't to say that the family of six who lives at Long Dream don't work their tails off—no one ever said farming is easy. But their lifestyle certainly appears to represent the type of pastoral ideal that has become so foreign to most of us. And it doesn't hurt that the heritage cattle raised here are likely the goshdarn cutest cows you'll ever meet.

Long Dream Farm is run by Krista and Andrew Abrahams and their four children ranging in age from young adult to young child. Everyone pitches in, and between the farm-stay guesthouse, free-range-egg production, heritage cattle breeding, and milking operations, there's plenty to keep them all busy. You'd hardly know it, though, from the leisurely farm tours Krista conducts for visitors. The tours last close to 2 hours and introduce visitors to the farm's many animals while showcasing the gorgeous topography of the 90-acre Long Dream property—a hilly, tree-dotted piece of land graced with natural ponds and creeks. The farm is laid out in a circular pattern around the main hill, with the family home at the top, the young livestock enclosures and barn placed closest to the house, and fields and pastures fanning out toward the base of the hill.

While the relatively mild climate in Placer County allows the animals of Long Dream to be outdoors year-round, the Abrahamses have chosen to raise hardy breeds of both cattle and chicken that thrive in the fluctuating temperatures of the Sierra Nevada foothills. The farm is home to approximately 1,200 pastured chickens that lay between 40 dozen and 70 dozen eggs a day, depending on the season. The youngest chicks hang out on the grassy area nearest the house, while the laying hens are divided among several chicken houses, each with plenty of outdoor space and its own rooster. The farm is also home to pigs, alpacas, emus, and turkeys. But the biggest stars here are the cows, mostly heritage breeds such as Scottish Highlands and Dexters, which are smaller than typical dairy cows and so furry and cute you'll be tempted to take one home as a pet. And that idea isn't so far-fetched; part of Long Dream's business is breeding and training well-socialized dairy cows to sell to homesteaders.

Even though most of the cows are raised for their milk, the Abrahamses keep the calves on their mothers and milk only once a day to cause less stress to the animals. The dairy cows are also allowed to roam the 90-acre farm, resting in the shade of the oak trees, munching on acorns and grazing on the abundant grass. The farm's fences are arranged to form an ingenious alley system that gives the herds access to more than 30 grazing pastures, which leads to a natural pattern of rotational

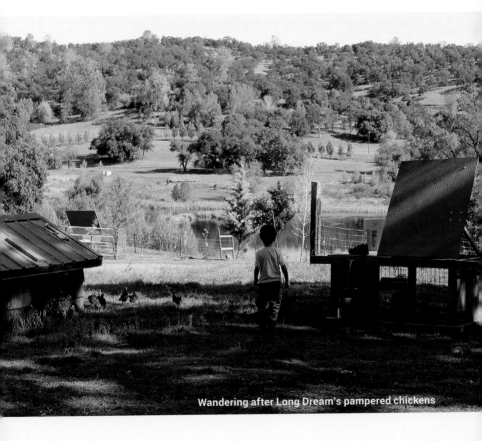

Wandering after Long Dream's pampered chickens

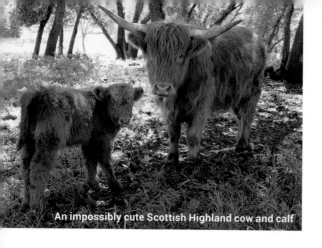
An impossibly cute Scottish Highland cow and calf

grazing, thereby ensuring that the grasslands are consistently rested and replenished to create a sustainable feeding loop.

While Krista's farm tours are unrushed and visitors are welcome to picnic on the grounds afterward, you may well find that you want to spend even more time at Long Dream. To that end, a very reasonably priced farm stay is offered in the four-bedroom, two-bathroom guesthouse, which has a fully equipped kitchen and comfortably sleeps eight people. Guests are welcome to help out with farm chores, if desired, or simply hike, swim (in the warm season), stargaze, play, and enjoy the breathtaking natural surroundings.

TIPS Krista or Andrew will provide directions to the farm when you schedule a visit, but it can still be a little hard to find and, depending on which direction you come from, could include a stretch of unpaved road. Don't be shy about asking for extremely detailed directions to ensure that you don't get turned around on the country roads. Also, touring the farm involves walking through animal pastures and crossing a creek that may be partially flooded by beaver dams, so wear shoes that you don't mind getting mucky.

4 PRESTON FARM AND WINERY

9282 W. Dry Creek Road, Healdsburg, CA 95448; 707-433-3372, prestonvineyards.com; open year-round

WHAT THEY OFFER Farm stand, picnicking, seasonal events, tasting

SONOMA COUNTY'S DRY CREEK VALLEY delivers the kind of imagery most people dream about when they think of California's wine country. Thousands of acres of lush grapevines climb into oak-covered hillsides with mountain redwood forests as a backdrop. This is pastoral landscape at its most picturesque. As you follow Dry Creek Road north from the 101 freeway, you'll periodically pass white picket signposts pointing toward what seems like dozens of wineries in every direction. And while many of them are surely worth visiting, particularly if you're an oenophile, one of the most notable is Preston of Dry Creek up in Geyserville. The family-owned winery founded in the 1970s has evolved from a conventional estate winery into a diversified organic farm. Today, you'll pass vegetable gardens and colorful chicken coops as you follow the long dirt road toward the winery's tasting room.

In their 40-plus years of experience growing on this land in the Russian River watershed, Preston's owners and farmers have spent a great deal of time getting to know their land and their soil. They've

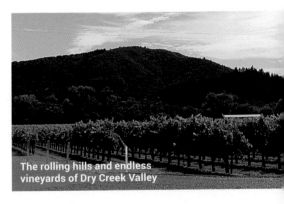

The rolling hills and endless vineyards of Dry Creek Valley

diversified so far beyond grapes that they now grow veggies, fruits, nuts, and grains and raise pastured sheep, chickens, and pigs. For anyone interested in learning more about any of their crops or livestock, the folks at Preston offer an incredibly comprehensive farming biography on their website; true agricultural wonks can even check out their soil map to get into the real nitty-gritty of what they grow and how they grow it.

Preston welcomes visitors seven days a week to its tasting room and farm store. The tasting room offers the expected assortment of reds, whites, and rosés, as well as estate-grown olive oil, olives, and fresh-baked bread. The diverse selection continues next door in the farm store, where you'll find seasonal produce, house-made vinegars, freshly laid eggs, and various pickled and fermented products. After sipping and sampling, visitors can enjoy the lovely picnic grounds surrounded by wildflower gardens or play on the bocce court. Guided tours of the farm and vineyards are offered exclusively to wine club members, but casual visitors are welcome to embark on a self-guided tour of the farm and gardens. Preston also hosts seasonal public events such as a harvest festival and holiday party, as well as regular farm dinners paired with its biodynamic wines.

NEARBY ATTRACTION Healdsburg SHED

Downtown Healdsburg is exactly the type of quaint city square you'd expect to find in Sonoma Valley wine country. Storefronts include cleverly named bakeries, upscale boutiques (for people and their pets), and restaurants offering fresh fare and patio dining. SHED may be downtown's unofficial flagship, as it combines a café, bakery, garden supply, pantry, and marketplace in one big, light-filled, industrial-chic space. It's pretty irresistible.

SHED also sells farming supplies, albeit at prices that would likely make "real" farmers scoff. But the offerings will appeal to hobby gardeners and aspiring urban homesteaders looking for a carefully edited selection of high-quality tools, along with some great books for guidance. A small outdoor area also offers plants and pottery for sale.

25 North St., Healdsburg, CA 95448; 707-431-7433, healdsburgshed.com

5 SOIL BORN FARMS

2140 Chase Drive, Rancho Cordova, CA 95670; 916-363-9685, soilborn.org; open year-round

WHAT THEY OFFER Apprenticeships, camps, classes and workshops, CSA (community-supported agriculture), farm stand, tours, volunteer opportunities

SOIL BORN FARMS' URBAN AGRICULTURE AND EDUCATION PROJECT has an enviably un-urban home on the scenic and historic 55-acre American River Ranch property in the Sacramento suburb of Rancho Cordova. The property is a veritable natural playground for kids and adults alike with its learning gardens, happy farm animals, campfire circles, children's play area, and walking trails leading to the river. The farm is open to visitors for self-guided tours Monday–Saturday, dawn–dusk and hosts events and classes throughout the year, as well as summer day camps. This accessibility stems from its founders' mission to bring sustainable farming practices and healthy food education to as many people as possible in the hopes of inspiring future urban farmers.

Interestingly enough, Soil Born began as a private, for-profit farm back in 2000. Shawn Harrison and Marco Franciosa were self-described young and inexperienced farmers with a shared dream and lots of ambition to reconnect urban dwellers with healthy, organically grown food. When Janet Whalen Zeller joined the team in 2002, they collectively decided to transform the farm into a nonprofit with an emphasis on promoting healthy eating and hands-on agricultural education in the Sacramento community. The farm's location on the American River Parkway, a protected 55-acre piece of land surrounded by urban and suburban development, also provides an excellent opportunity to integrate environmental stewardship into their programs by taking advantage of the diverse and beautiful natural landscape.

Casual visitors to the farm are encouraged to grab a map near the parking lot and embark on a self-guided tour. Highly informative signs are posted throughout the property, detailing the history of the land and

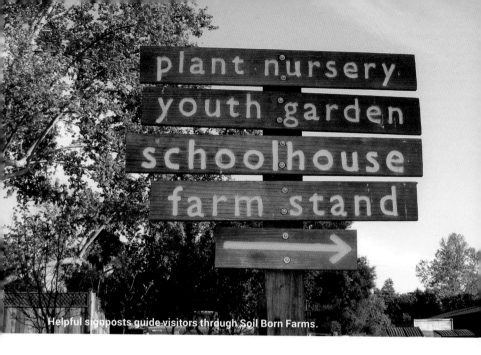

Helpful signposts guide visitors through Soil Born Farms.

the organic farming practices currently in place, from seed starting to native-plant restoration to composting. Particularly interesting are the native-pollinator garden, the youth garden and, of course, the resident farm animals, which include cows, pigs, sheep, and chickens. For little ones, a thoughtfully designed playground includes natural features like tree stumps, stepping-stones, and logs, as well as a towering climbing structure. The site is also home to an outdoor classroom, schoolhouse, and farmhouse kitchen used for summer day camps.

Soil Born Farms is relatively quiet during the winter, even though the property is open to visitors. Things really get hopping May–November, when the American River Ranch farm stand is open every Saturday and the farm hosts regular public events and classes on topics such as water-wise gardening, backyard chicken-keeping, herbal medicine, solar cooking, permaculture, and birding. Like all nonprofit organizations, Soil Born also welcomes volunteers to help out in all aspects of running the farm. Opportunities may include working in the garden or applying much-needed skills in areas like carpentry and culinary arts.

For those students who want to take their farming education to the next level, apprenticeships are also offered at Soil Born Farms. The first-year program is a full-time, eight-month-long position that explores all aspects of sustainable food production. Apprentices reside at the American River Ranch in canvas platform tents with access to the indoor kitchen, shower, and shared living room. First-year graduates are invited to apply for the second-year apprenticeship, which involves more advanced training and deepening of skills based on the student's particular interests, and may even provide the opportunity to take over management of the Farm on Hurley Way, a separate 1-acre operation run by Soil Born.

TIP The turn for Soil Born can be easy to miss, and the farm's sign is small. As you're driving up Octavia Way, look for a narrow road to the left before you reach the parking entrance for Hagan Community Park. Soil Born is down that road and has its own small dirt parking lot.

---

6 TERRA SAVIA

14160 Mountain House Road, Hopland, CA 95449; 707-744-1114, terrasavia.com; open year-round

WHAT THEY OFFER Lodging, special events, tasting

TERRA SAVIA WINERY IS A LOT COOLER AND FUNKIER than any winery has a right to be. Overseen by husband-and-wife team Yvonne Hall and Jurg Fischer, this 35-acre property in Hopland is a combination winery, olive oil mill, and art gallery, with some heirloom tomato crops, chickens, rescued pigeons, and a guesthouse rental thrown in, to boot. Yes, they do it all here, but the atmosphere is nonetheless laid-back and pleasant—just what you'd expect to find in rustically beautiful Mendocino County.

The first things you'll notice when you enter the main facility are the giant stainless steel olive auger-washer and three-wheeled granite crusher. The olive oil and wine-tasting bars, which are hand-carved from

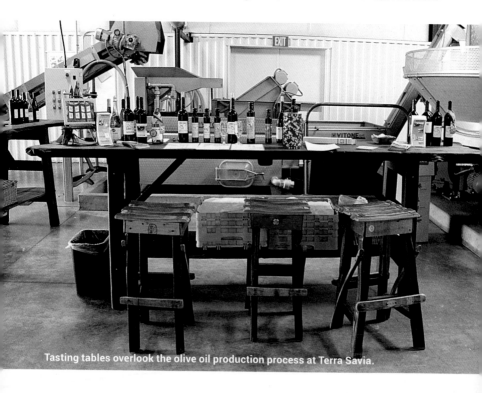

Tasting tables overlook the olive oil production process at Terra Savia.

old-growth redwood with stools sculpted from repurposed wine barrels, are placed directly in front of the machines, giving the manufacturing process pride of place in a place that does it all, from growing to processing to bottling to labeling. In addition to growing olives to make their own extra-virgin olive oils, Terra Savia presses and bottles olive oil for hundreds of growers—from boutique to well known—many of which are on display in wooden racks in the olive mill.

Terra Savia's owners are usually on hand to walk visitors through the entire production process and explain what each of the impressive giant stainless steel machines does. The state-of-the-art olive mill features both the granite crusher for clients who want their EVOO to have a smoother, more buttery taste, and a blade crusher—used for Terra Savia's own label, which produces a bolder flavor profile. The

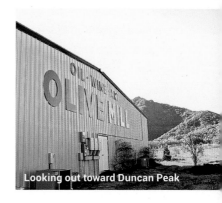
Looking out toward Duncan Peak

malaxer begins the initial separation process, in which the oil rises to the top of the ground-up olive paste. Stainless steel tubes then carry the paste to the decanter, or centrifuge, which further separates the solids from the liquids. The vegetative water and oil are then carried to the separator, which spins very fast to finally separate the oil from the water. Because Terra Savia mainly produces unfiltered olive oil, the oils are typically then left to settle for two months before being drained off the sediment and bottled.

Terra Savia is an incredibly green operation and strives to produce as little waste as possible in the production process. To that end, the olive solids are composted in partnership with the city, the vegetative water is used to oil gravel roads and keep the dust down, and the sediment that is left at the end of the process is sold to beauty manufacturers to be made into soap and other products. The company is also certified organic, as well as "fish friendly," meaning that any runoff or by-products of the manufacturing process are carefully managed so as not to disturb the delicate ecosystem of the nearby creeks. All of Terra Savia's buildings are solar-powered, and the water used to irrigate the vineyards comes from a natural spring on the property.

In addition to the tasting tables inside the main facility, Terra Savia has a private tasting room built of reclaimed wood with stained glass accents. A great spot for wedding parties (nearby Campovida, page 8, is a popular wedding location), the little cabin has a wood-burning stove and a hammock, as well as a deck covered with a grape arbor—guests are encouraged to pluck and eat the heirloom table grapes that grow here in season. You'd be hard-pressed to find a more rustically charming setting for wine tasting. And for those who'd like to stay here even longer—and who wouldn't?—a two-bedroom guesthouse at the base of Duncan Peak at the rear of the property offers all of the comforts of home, including a full kitchen, central air and heat, a barbecue grill, an enclosed yard, a hot tub, and an aboveground swimming pool, in a gorgeous, secluded setting. The most alluring perk of staying in this vacation rental is the access it affords to the nearby pond house, a towering reclaimed-wood building that looks like it sprang from the pages of a children's picture book and features a cozy nook and a roomy deck looking out over Terra Savia's natural spring and vineyards.

ADDITIONAL FARMS IN THE AREA

Apple Hill
Visit applehill.com for a list of all locations and for directions.

This collection of more than 50 ranches near Placerville has been a popular family apple-picking and recreation destination since 1964. The farms and ranches are open seasonally for pick-your-own apples, cherries, blueberries, pumpkins, and more, and many locations also sell treats such as fresh-pressed cider and pie. You'll also find flower and Christmas tree farms, along with spas and wineries.

Capay Organic
23804 CA 16, Capay, CA 95607; 530-796-0730, capayorganic.com

Capay Organic has been farming organically since 1976 and now grows over 130 varieties of fruits and vegetables on 500 acres of land. The farm supplies produce to local farmers markets, restaurants, and stores, as well as to subscribers to the popular Farm Fresh to You produce delivery service throughout California. Capay also hosts public events throughout the year, including farm tours, holiday celebrations, 5Ks, and farm dinners.

Emandal
16500 Hearst Post Office Road, Willits, CA 95490; 707-459-5439, emandal.com

This peaceful farm retreat on the Eel River near Willits in Mendocino County may be best known for its summer Family Camp, which draws the same families back year after year for a total escape into the natural world. Rates include three made-from-scratch meals daily and activities like swimming, hiking, stargazing, games, and farm chores. Emandal also hosts open work days and art retreats throughout the year and offers lodging in its redwood cabins, farmhouse, and bunkhouse to private groups and individuals.

Full Belly Farm

16090 CR 43, Guinda, CA 95637; 530-796-2214, fullbellyfarm.com

Full Belly Farm is a certified organic, socially responsible farm that offers a popular CSA for Bay Area residents. The farm may be best known for its annual "Hoes Down" harvest festival, a weekend-long event that offers educational workshops, family-friendly activities, dancing, and an overall good time. The beautiful 350-acre piece of land is also open for occasional public farm tours, farm dinners, and school field trips.

Grange Farm School

Near Ukiah, California; 860-670-7146, grangefarmschool.org. Call or visit the website for directions.

Founded with the purpose of "educating the whole farmer," the Grange Farm School is located on the site of Ridgewood Ranch, just off US 101 between Ukiah and Willits. Offerings include a three-month residential program (a.k.a. "farm school") for aspiring farmers as well as weekend workshops on topics such as pruning, constructing a cold frame, and the business of sustainable agriculture.

Jug Handle Creek Farm and Nature Center

15501 N. CA 1, Caspar, CA 95420; 707-964-1825, jughandlecreekfarm.com

Jug Handle Creek Farm is a nature education center that offers after-school programs and summer day camps for students, as well as lodging for overnight visitors, in the campground, cabins, or historic Victorian farmhouse. The coastal 39-acre property encompasses forests and meadows, as well as community gardens and a native plants nursery. The grounds are part of the Jug Handle State Reserve and offer easy access to hiking the historically and geologically significant trail known as The Ecological Staircase, a terraced land formation where each level is 100,000 years older than the next.

Mar Vista Cottages

35101 S. CA 1, Gualala, CA 95445; 877-855-3522, marvistamendocino.com

These restored historic cottages on the Mendocino Coast give guests the opportunity to simultaneously experience farm life and a beautiful coastal getaway at Anchor Bay. The twelve cottages that dot the property can accommodate anyone from individuals looking for quiet seclusion to families with young children who will enjoy gathering eggs from the hens and frolicking through the orchard and gardens. Guests are invited to gather ingredients from the edible garden to prepare meals in their own cottage kitchens.

Philo Apple Farm

18501 Greenwood Road, Philo, CA 95466; 707-895-2333,
philoapplefarm.com

Whether you simply stop by the farm stand for a glass of cold, fresh-pressed apple juice or decide to splurge and stay at the inn to enjoy a weekend of cooking classes, farm life, and incredible meals, Philo Apple Farm is worth a visit. While you're in the area, check out nearby Boonville as well. The small town invented the now almost-extinct Boontling dialect and is home to Farmhouse Mercantile (farmhouse 128.com), a modern-day general store run by the same family as the Apple Farm, as well as the Anderson Valley Brewing Company brewhouse and taproom (avbc.com).

Quivira Vineyards

4900 W. Dry Creek Road, Healdsburg, CA 95448; 707-431-8333,
quivirawine.com

Located just a few miles south of Preston Farm and Winery (see page 17) on West Dry Creek Road, Quivira Vineyards is another winery devoted to biodynamic farming methods (see page 153 for more on the subject). Visitors are welcome to explore the 1-acre garden during the winery's daily tasting-room hours, and guided estate tours are also offered.

River Hill Farm

13500 Cement Hill Road, Nevada City, CA 95959; 530-263-1886,
riverhillfarm.com

River Hill is one of the many local farms that supply ingredients to Three Forks Bakery (see next page); here they grow a diverse range of organic crops on 10 acres of land with plans to grow larger while still serving the local community. The farm stand is open once a week from May or June until November, and visitors are invited to look around and enjoy the farm's beautiful setting overlooking the Yuba River.

Scott River Ranch

1138 E. Callahan Road, Etna, CA 96027; 877-542-1802, scottriverranch.com

This family-run, grass-fed, organic, Animal Welfare Approved beef ranch is located way up north near the tiny town of Etna in Siskiyou County. Because the proprietors hold the firm belief that beef is best enjoyed when you know where it came from, the ranch is pretty much always open to visitors. If you make it up to the area, call or e-mail ahead of time and let them know you'd like to take a look around.

Three Forks Bakery and Brewing Co.

211 Commercial St., Nevada City, CA 95959; 530-470-8333,
threeforksnc.com

Three Forks isn't a farm; it's a restaurant. But because the owners,
chefs, bakers, brewers and butchers here are so committed to using
ingredients from local farmers and making everything themselves
from scratch, it offers an incredible taste of all things local and
delicious in the Sierra Nevada foothills. They even give their coffee
grounds, food waste, and spent beer grain back to local farmers to
feed their animals. Come in for a cold microbrew and an unforgettable
thin-crust pizza, and be sure to save room for dessert—all of the
pastries here taste incredible as well. Walk it off afterward by exploring Nevada City's almost implausibly quaint historic district.

Wakamatsu Tea and Silk Colony Farm

941 Cold Springs Road, Placerville, CA 95667; 530-621-1224,
arconservancy.org

A cultural-heritage site overseen by the American River Conservancy,
Wakamatsu incorporates a rich and expansive wildlife habitat, histor-
ical buildings and landmarks, and working sustainable-agricultural
operations. The 272-acre property includes a lake, ponds, wetlands,
and woodlands, along with fertile farming soil; the South Fork Farm
CSA and family-owned Free Hand Farm currently operate on the site.
Public tours of the farm are held monthly, and private tours can be
arranged as well. The conservancy also regularly hosts workshops
and welcomes volunteers.

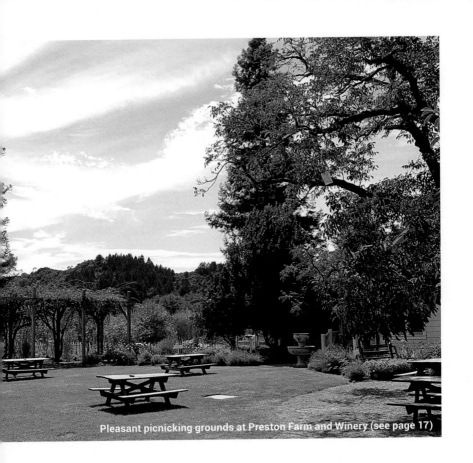

Pleasant picnicking grounds at Preston Farm and Winery (see page 17)

San Francisco
BAY AREA

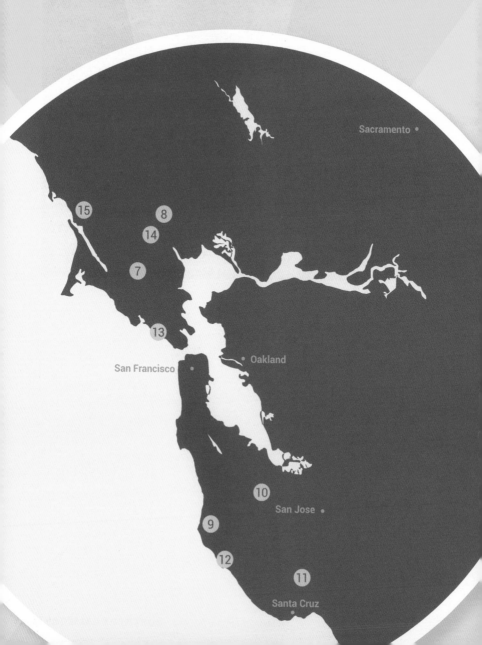

Sacramento

15

8

14

7

13

Oakland

San Francisco

10

San Jose

9

12

11

Santa Cruz

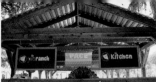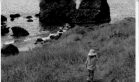

FARMS TO VISIT IN THE
SAN FRANCISCO BAY AREA

7 COW TRACK RANCH

5730 Nicasio Valley Road, Nicasio, CA 94946; 415-662-2321, cowtrackranch.com; open year-round. Call or e-mail cowtrackranch@gmail.com for detailed directions.

WHAT THEY OFFER Event venue, hiking, lodging

IF THE TRAFFIC, AMBIENT NOISE, and—let's face it—people in your everyday life have you craving solitude and isolation, the Bunk House at Cow Track Ranch fills the bill. Located in the town of Nicasio in Marin County, the 468-acre ranch is reached via almost 1.5 miles of unpaved road and surrounded on all sides by rolling hills populated almost

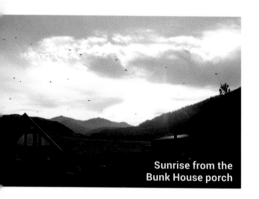

Sunrise from the Bunk House porch

exclusively by contented cows and native wildlife. Liz and Bruce Daniels have owned and operated Cow Track Ranch for nearly 30 years and, as a nod to the growing interest in agritourism, renovated the "bunk house" next door to their main house and started renting it out to guests in 2011.

The Bunk House has all the rustic charm you'd expect in a setting like this. It sleeps up to five with a king-size bed in the master bedroom and another king and a twin bed up in the sleeping loft. Furnishings are comfortable, a wood-burning stove keeps things cozy, and the small kitchen is equipped with the basic cooking tools and utensils you'll need to make your own meals. During the growing season, guests are welcome to pick their own produce from the adjacent garden that Liz maintains.

Kids will be delighted with the loft and even find an assortment of children's books up there. But parents of toddlers should be advised that this house is by no means childproof—large gaps between the railings of the loft and knickknacks galore make this dwelling best suited to grown-ups and older children. Part of the pleasure of staying in the

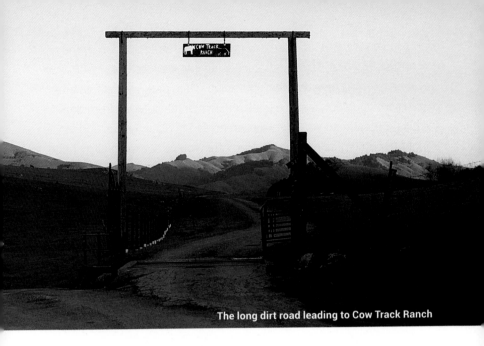

The long dirt road leading to Cow Track Ranch

Bunk House is the absence of distractions. There's no television or Wi-Fi. Your best indoor entertainment will come from reading (you'll find plenty of books on the shelves) and watching "cow TV" through the cabin's many windows.

Despite the fact that Liz and Bruce's home is just outside your back door, you have a sense of total privacy in the Bunk House. That said, Liz is just a knock away if you need anything. When you do see Liz, she'll put you immediately at ease; she has a laid-back drawl and "no worries" attitude that belies how hard she and Bruce work to keep this nearly 500-acre ranch running, run their horse-veterinarian business, host special events, and act as innkeepers, to boot. Bruce, meanwhile, is likely to lay pretty low during your visit, but if you do find a chance to chat, it will be a treat to hear him talk about the vagaries of cattle ranching, while at the same time expressing a deep appreciation and awe for the beauty of the land he has the pleasure of overseeing.

Cow Track Ranch's property runs from the lush grassland of the Nicasio Valley up into live oak–shaded hillsides, and hiking its trails offers panoramic views of the surrounding hills and ranches. Because the location is so picturesque, the ranch is popular for weddings and other special events. If you want to start the day off right, rise early and follow the trail north of the Bunk House that leads up into the hills—the 1,000-foot elevation gain will get your heart pumping. Then park yourself on one of the giant boulders near the peak and watch the sun rise from behind the hills. Guaranteed you'll feel as serene as the Black Angus and Texas Longhorn cattle grazing down below. After you've soaked it all in, head back down to your cozy abode, brew a pot of coffee, and enjoy munching on the delicious pastries from Bovine Bakery in Point Reyes Station that Liz has so thoughtfully left for you in the kitchen as you watch the cows peacefully eating their own breakfast just outside your window.

NEARBY ATTRACTION Point Reyes Station

Situated as it is among a treasure trove of small farms, the coastal town of Point Reyes Station is a tiny mecca for foodies and nature lovers alike. The nearby protected lands of the Point Reyes National Seashore offer endless opportunities for hiking, camping, biking, kayaking, and other outdoor adventures, while the picturesque downtown is home to the original location of the immensely popular Cowgirl Creamery, located in a restored hay barn at Tomales Bay Foods. Here you can order delicious sandwiches and salads or pick up a loaf of bread and a bottle of wine to go with your fromage blanc and simply enjoy the pleasant nearby picnic area. While you're here, check out the goods at Toby's Feed Barn, a combination farm supply store, farmers market, yoga studio, coffee bar, art gallery, and gift shop. Also, be sure to pick up a pastry or an entire pie at Bovine Bakery, where the buttery baked goods are unforgettable. Everything in Point Reyes Station is located within a couple of blocks, so park the car and go exploring.

Shoreline Highway (CA 1) and Fourth Street,
Point Reyes Station, CA 94956

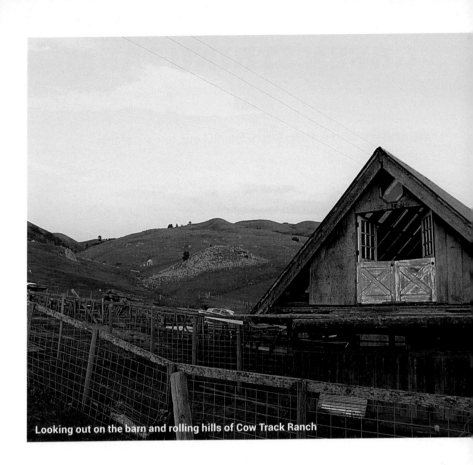

Looking out on the barn and rolling hills of Cow Track Ranch

8 GREEN STRING FARM

3571 Old Adobe Road, Petaluma, CA 94954; 707-778-7500, greenstringfarm.com; open year-round

WHAT THEY OFFER Farm stand, picnicking, tours, training and internships

IF IT WEREN'T FOR THE FARM STAND OUT FRONT, Green String Farm could almost be mistaken for a wildlife preserve at first glance. An abundance of birds twitter and flit about in the marshy area near the parking lot, and acres and acres of what appears to be uncultivated land interspersed with grapevines stretches up the hillsides into the middle distance.

This is by design. Green String's founders, Bob Cannard and Fred Cline, are devoted to a farming method that is generally referred to as "beyond organic." The basic premise can be summed up as follows: soil is a living organism; feed it well and it will be able to take care of itself. There's a more scientific explanation, of course, having to do with microorganisms and microbes, but all a layperson really needs to know is that healthy plants come from healthy soil, and healthy soil is built with natural fortifiers such as compost tea, crushed oyster shells, and volcanic ash. Build up the soil with these completely natural amendments, and you forgo the need for chemical fertilizers and pesticides.

Weeds, too, are welcome at Green String Farm. In between crop plantings, native weeds and other plants are allowed to grow in the fields and then die back into the soil to fortify it further, functioning much like a cover crop. The farm also employs other sustainable methods to keep the land healthy. A herd of sheep weed the vineyards and trim the grapevines (but not when the grapes are ripe, of course; otherwise they'd consume the whole expensive crop). Native plants and beehives attract pollinators and other beneficial insects, and diligent interplanting and crop rotation ensure that no single crop is ever allowed to deplete the soil of its inherent attributes.

Green String's farmers' painstakingly sustainable methods don't translate to the highest profits possible, but the reward is the knowledge that they are true stewards of the land, keeping these 350 acres strong and productive for generations to come. Another huge upside is the quality of the produce. Green String is a major provider of fruits and vegetables to Alice Waters' famed Chez Panisse, as well as Thomas Keller's French Laundry.

But you don't have to be a renowned chef to enjoy the bounty of Green String Farm. The farm stand is open seven days a week, offering seasonal produce, as well as homemade flour; grass-fed meats from a sister property in Red Bluff; Green String's own honey, olive oil, and preserves; and cheeses from local purveyors. The farm stand is a staple of the local Petaluma community—the same customers come in every week; children enjoy the playhouse out back, families picnic outside,

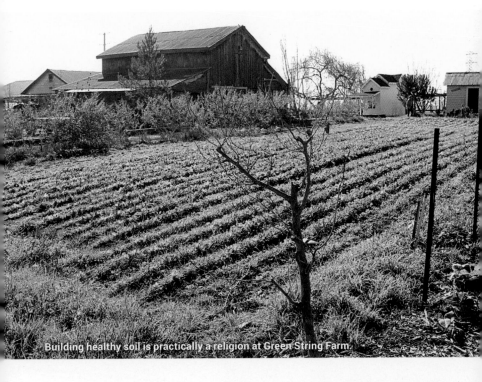
Building healthy soil is practically a religion at Green String Farm.

and shoppers enjoy picking out beautiful fresh produce in the homey shop, where a wood-burning stove keeps things cozy on chilly days and, if you're lucky, a Patsy Cline album is playing on the record player.

In addition to employing the Green String method on their own farm, the owners also operate the Green String Institute, a six-week internship that teaches participants the beyond-organic method of farming, along with every other aspect of farming and animal husbandry they'd need to know to start their own sustainable farming operations. And for those who simply want to get an overview of sustainable farming methods, Green String offers free community tours every Saturday at noon (call to confirm), as well as school field trips and private tours by appointment.

NEARBY ATTRACTION Petaluma Seed Bank

Located in an impressive 1920s former bank in Petaluma's lovely and historic downtown area, the Petaluma Seed Bank is home to Baker Creek Heirloom Seed Company's West Coast location. Gardening enthusiasts can browse more than 1,500 varieties of heirloom seeds, as well as gardening tools, books, and food and gift items, and marvel at the huge arched windows and high hammered-metal ceilings of this grand old Victorian building.

199 Petaluma Blvd. N., Petaluma, CA 94952; 707-773-1336, rareseeds.com

9 HARLEY FARMS

205 North St., Pescadero, CA 94060; 650-879-0480, harleyfarms.com;
open year-round

WHAT THEY OFFER Farm stand, gift shop, picnicking, special events,
tasting, tours

THE TINY COASTAL TOWN OF PESCADERO, just about halfway between
San Francisco and Santa Cruz, may be best known for its proximity
to Año Nuevo State Park, where thousands of elephant seals can be
observed lounging on the rocks and shore year-round. But despite its
blissfully bucolic natural surroundings, Pescadero has more to offer
than just nature hikes and seal-gazing. Stage Road, the town's historic,
two-block main drag, is home to the Pescadero Country Store, where
you can order excellent pizza from a wood-burning oven, and Duarte's
Tavern, which was established in 1894 with a barrel of whiskey hauled
up from Santa Cruz. Yes, despite its diminutive size, this town warrants
more than just a pit stop. To that end, charming and comfortable
overnight accommodations can be had at the Pescadero Creek Inn
(see "Nearby Lodging," page 41).

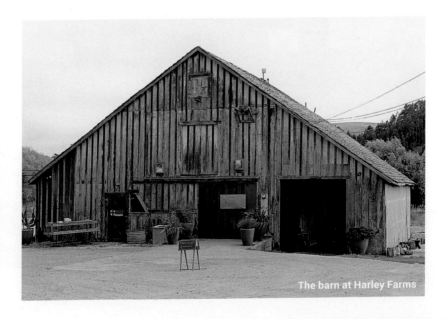

The barn at Harley Farms

But the main attraction that draws visitors to Pescadero is Harley Farms Goat Dairy and its award-winning chèvre, fromage blanc, ricotta, and feta cheeses. The restored 1910 cow dairy was transformed into a farmstead goat dairy by veteran farmer Dee Harley in 2007 and is now home to about 200 Alpine goats that enjoy roaming 12 acres of pasture. Casual visitors are welcome to stroll around the farm to see the goats and llamas (that protect the goats from predators). Spring is the best time of year to visit, as you're likely to see some baby goats frolicking in Tony's Pen. The pleasantly rustic farm shop is open daily and sells the aforementioned cheeses, along with jams, jellies, and the Harley Farms Bath and Body collection of soaps, oils, balms, and lotions. Perhaps the most interesting item on offer is FarmPaint, a completely nontoxic, bio-degradable, VOC-free house paint made from goat's milk and available in nine vibrant colors. Above the shop is a picturesque hayloft used to host farm dinners and other events; it features magnificent, oversize carved wooden chairs and a long fir table fit for royalty, along with a balcony overlooking the vegetable garden below.

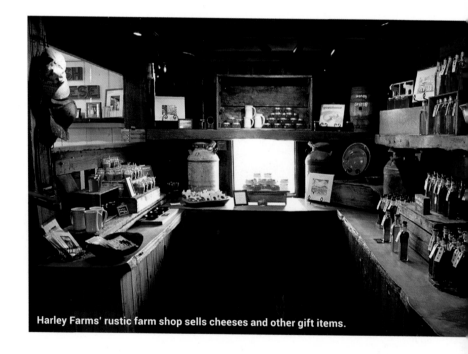

Harley Farms' rustic farm shop sells cheeses and other gift items.

At the Pescadero Creek Inn, attractive and homey accommodations are available within walking distance of Harley Farms and all the businesses and attractions of Stage Road. Friendly innkeepers Ken and Penny renovated this century-old farmhouse with comfort and hospitality in mind and now offer guests their choice of three rooms or a separate garden cottage, each with its own distinct furnishings and features. Charming touches such as feather mattresses and antique claw-foot tubs lend a relaxing, old-fashioned vibe to the inn, and guests are invited to mix and mingle over morning coffee in front of the old stone fireplace in the front parlor. The grounds are lovely, as well, with meandering garden paths overlooking Pescadero Creek. If you'd like a little more privacy or are staying with a child, try to book the standalone Garden Cottage, which features a separate daybed, private deck, and view of the garden.

393 Stage Road, Pescadero, CA 94060; 650-879-1898, pescaderocreekinn.com

If you'd like to gain a deeper understanding of how a farmstead goat dairy works, book a spot on one of Harley's Goat Tours, which are offered almost every weekend. The 2-hour tours feature plenty of hands-on activity and cheese tasting, so come hungry and wear farm-appropriate attire, including sturdy closed-toe shoes. You'll meet the goats, who are separated by age on different areas of the farm, and follow the entire process, from the milking shed to the dairy, where their milk is transformed into curd and, finally, gourmet cheeses. Afterward, you're invited to picnic on the picturesque grounds. Separate tours are offered for families with children and for adults only, and school field trips and corporate retreats may be booked here as well.

NEARBY ATTRACTION AND LODGING
Pigeon Point Lighthouse

As you head south on CA 1 from Pescadero to Santa Cruz, which is referred to as Cabrillo Highway on this stretch, you'll pass U-pick farms and roadside farm stands. It's an amazingly idyllic segment of highway, so plan to take your time on the journey so you can make stops for freshly picked produce and gorgeous ocean views from atop the bluffs. The stately Pigeon Point Lighthouse is just off CA 1 about 5 miles south of Pescadero Creek Road. This popular whale-watching spot is also home to a hostel offering affordable lodging on a beautiful, historic site.

210 Pigeon Point Road, Pescadero, CA 94060; 650-879-0633, norcalhostels.org

TIP If you're not visiting with children of your own, you may want to book one of the adults-only weekend tours so there are fewer distractions. And if you decide to picnic on the grounds, plan to supplement your provisions with some cheese, jams, and jellies from the shop so you can get a taste of what Harley has to offer. Also note that pets are not allowed on the farm.

10 HIDDEN VILLA

26870 Moody Road, Los Altos Hills, CA 94022; 650-949-8650, hiddenvilla.org.
Open year-round but may be closed to visitors during summer programs;
visit the website to confirm.

WHAT THEY OFFER Camps, CSA, hiking, lodging, special events,
tours, training and internships, volunteer opportunities

HIDDEN VILLA HAS A RICH AND IMPRESSIVE HISTORY. Activists
Josephine and Frank Duveneck purchased this choice parcel of land in
beautiful Los Altos Hills (the heart of what is now Silicon Valley) back
in 1924 with a vision for social reform. Their altruistic nature and dedicated efforts produced the first multiracial summer camp in 1945 and
an early environmental education program in 1970.

Today, the nonprofit continues to make education its first priority. Hidden Villa's tagline is "Inspiring a just and sustainable future through our
programs, land and legacy." And it has a lot of land to work with: 1,600
acres. Much of that acreage is devoted to wilderness preservation, and
the property features miles of scenic hiking trails open to the public,
ranging from relatively flat, cool, and shady to steep and challeng-
ing. Pick up a comprehensive trail map with recommended hikes and
descriptions at the visitor center upon arrival.

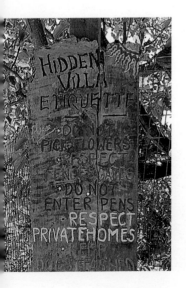

A small portion of the property—about
8 acres—has been cultivated for agriculture, and that number can drop during
drought conditions. Hidden Villa's produce is available for sale at the Los Altos
farmers market and to local families sub-
scribed to its CSA program. In addition to
fields of fruits and veggies, Hidden Villa
keeps animals for teaching purposes. The
menagerie includes pigs, chickens, goats,
sheep, and cows. Animal welfare is a given
on this organic farm, and all livestock
enjoy access to open pasture.

The property is usually closed to visitors during the summer months because this is when it caters exclusively to summer campers, offering extensive scholarships and financial aid to make outdoor education available to economically disadvantaged youth. Much of this largesse can be attributed to the generosity and deep pockets of the organization's Silicon Valley benefactors. Day camp and sleep-away camp are offered for kids ages 6–17, giving campers hands-on farming and animal husbandry experience, along with an intense focus on social and environmental justice. Camp facilitators are devoted to providing a safe space for multicultural students to explore age-appropriate themes of race, class, and body image to help them build self-esteem, leadership abilities, and compassion. Hidden Villa also offers school programs in environmental education throughout the year, including field trips for younger students and leadership training and service-learning projects for teens.

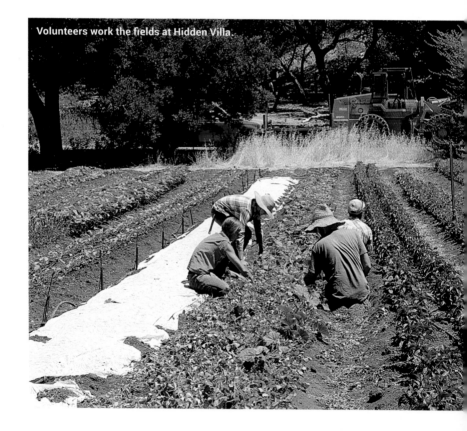

Volunteers work the fields at Hidden Villa.

Public programs for adults and families include lectures, hands-on workshops, and other classes and events. Guided tours of the farm are also open to the public and take place on weekends. Visit the website to see a calendar of events and to sign up.

Hidden Villa also welcomes volunteers—indeed, volunteer labor is integral to the farm's success, with more than 1,000 people helping each year. Many of the day laborers are there for corporate retreats, but individual volunteers also make up a huge part of the workforce. Short-term, drop-in volunteers are welcome, and there are also opportunities to make an ongoing commitment and become a part of the Hidden Villa family. Volunteer responsibilities may include trail maintenance, guiding farm tours, organic gardening, leading community programs, or even administrative assistance, and the appropriate training is provided for all tasks and positions.

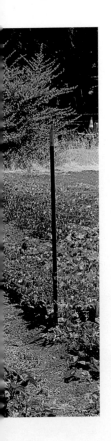

There are also a few rental properties on the land. Lodging is available in the historic Hidden Villa Hostel or at Josephine's Retreat, a cozy one-bedroom wooden cabin ideal for a romantic getaway. The property's Dana Center and historic Duveneck House are available for special events and corporate retreats but do not offer overnight accommodations.

11 LOVE APPLE FARMS

2317 Vine Hill Road, Santa Cruz, CA 95065; 831-588-3801, loveapplefarms.com.
Open to the public most weekends, but call ahead to confirm. Visit the website
for a schedule of classes and events. Detailed driving directions: tinyurl.com
/loveapplefarms.

WHAT THEY OFFER Apprenticeships, classes and workshops,
farm stand, special events, tours

TUCKED INTO A VERDANT VALLEY about halfway between Los Gatos
and Santa Cruz, Love Apple Farms is the very picture of what many
people probably dream about when they think of starting up their own
farm in coastal California. The property encompasses 22 acres, but
only a few acres have been cultivated, and the untouched surrounding
woodland of oaks, firs, and redwoods provides a stunning backdrop to
the farm's tidy terraced, raised-bed gardens. The productive and picturesque operation is overseen by Cynthia Sandberg, an avid gardener and

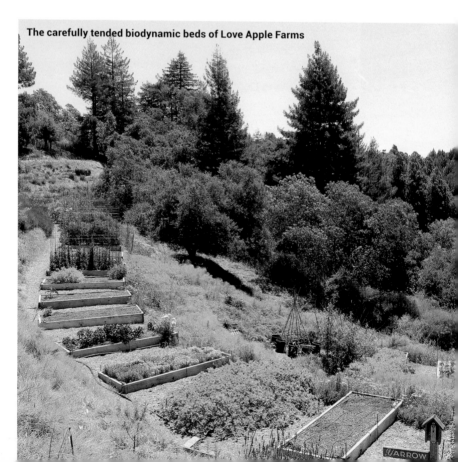

The carefully tended biodynamic beds of Love Apple Farms

former trial attorney who made the switch to full-time farming in 2000 with a tomato fruit stand in Ben Lomond. Cynthia moved Love Apple to its current home in 2010 and achieved biodynamic certification through the Demeter Association in 2012.

Love Apple's commitment to biodynamic agriculture involves practices that go beyond basic organic farming methods, nurturing a relationship between the soil, plants, and animals so that they form a fully integrated, self-nourishing system. This includes creating specific homeopathic herbal and mineral preparations that are added to the compost, and determining the planting schedule according to the astrological calendar. And while the process may sound a little labyrinthine to those unfamiliar with it, the philosophy is grounded in the sound and simple premise that plant pests and diseases are most effectively controlled when the entire farm organism, from soil to plant,

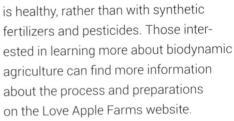

is healthy, rather than with synthetic fertilizers and pesticides. Those interested in learning more about biodynamic agriculture can find more information about the process and preparations on the Love Apple Farms website.

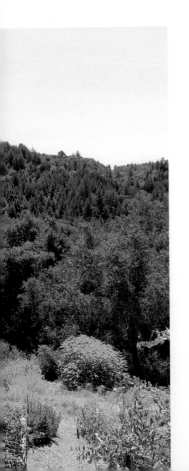

Proponents of biodynamic methods swear that these methods not only preserve the health of the land and soil but produce superior crops, as well, and the practice is catching on among many sustainable growers throughout the state. However, Love Apple is one of only a few certified biodynamic farms in California that offer public tours and educational programs. Docent-led tours happen once a month, and year-round workshops cover a wide range of topics, including canning and preserving, baking, cheese making, beekeeping, drip irrigation, composting, and vermiculture, to name just a few. In addition to agricultural education, Love Apple Farms grows hundreds of varieties of fruits, vegetables, edible flowers, and herbs exclusively for Manresa restaurant (manresarestaurant.com) in Los Gatos. Manresa's executive chef David Kinch is actively involved with Love Apple, and the restaurant's scraps are used to make compost, creating a closed-loop system between the farm and the restaurant.

Casual visitors are welcome on weekends to walk around the grounds and visit the farm stand, which sells the farm's homemade pickles and preserves, along with cheese-making supplies, seeds, seedlings, gardening books, and organic fertilizers. Love Apple also hosts beautiful al fresco farm dinners every couple of months or so—find a full schedule and pricing for all workshops, tours, and events on the website. The farm also offers an apprenticeship program, which includes on-site lodging with all the comforts of home (as opposed to a tent or yurt, as at other farm apprenticeship programs); excellent food; and, of course, a comprehensive education in biodynamic farming.

TIP For insurance purposes, visitors to the farm are asked to wear closed-toe shoes.

12 PIE RANCH

2080 Cabrillo Highway, Pescadero, CA 94060; 650-879-0995, pieranch.org; open year-round

WHAT THEY OFFER Apprenticeships, CSA, farm stand, special events, tours, training and internships, volunteer opportunities

BACK IN 2002, FOUNDING PARTNERS Nancy Vail, Jered Lawson, and Karen Heisler named this farm Pie Ranch for the triangular shape of their original 14-acre parcel (it has since expanded to 27 acres). Today, the name has taken on greater meaning. As they explain it, "Pie Ranch is a place for 'pie in the sky' idealistic thinking to guide social change, such as helping an urban school source local produce for their cafeteria, or a neighborhood to get their 'slice of the pie' to ensure access to high-quality fresh, locally grown foods." Almost equally important: They make really, really good pie.

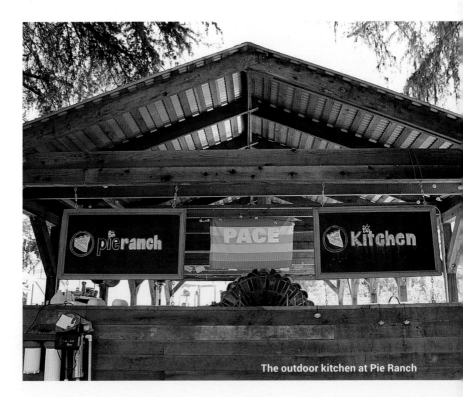

The outdoor kitchen at Pie Ranch

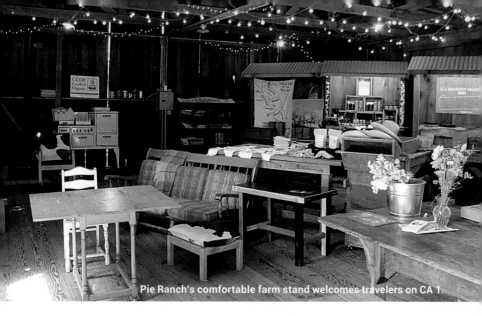

Pie Ranch's comfortable farm stand welcomes travelers on CA 1.

The primary focus at Pie Ranch is building a healthier food system through youth education and empowerment. They've partnered with high schools throughout the Bay Area to offer a series of field trips to build an ongoing education in farming and sustainable food production, from crops to cattle. Many high school students go on to participate in HomeSlice, the food systems internship program, which offers an education in culinary arts, sustainable agriculture, and community organizing for the sake of a healthier, more just food system.

Pie Ranch also provides training for adults. The Emerging Farmers Program offers both yearlong apprenticeships and summer internships. Living conditions for both programs are rustic—participants stay on the property and have access to an outdoor kitchen, bathroom, and shower. Apprentices lodge in either yurts or the historic house on the property, while interns pitch their own tents on the land. In addition to a monthly stipend, all participants get to enjoy all the farm-fresh produce they can eat (along with basic staples for preparing their own food). Although the internship is open to anyone interested in learning more about farming, apprentices must have spent at least one season working on a farm already. Both programs offer experience and education in all aspects of farming, including planting, weeding, irrigation, animal husbandry, working with youth, and direct marketing through the farm stand and CSA program.

If you'd like to get your hands dirty at the ranch without making a long-term commitment, attend one of Pie Ranch's scheduled work days and barn dances. You'll get to be a farmhand for the afternoon, helping out with whatever needs to be done that day, and then take an optional tour of the ranch. The real fun starts in the evening, with a live band, dancing, and a potluck dinner. This family-friendly party provides a great opportunity to cut loose, eat some great homemade food, and enjoy the company of the Pie Ranch farmers and other members of the community. Visit the website to find out when the next event is scheduled and to RSVP.

Of course, Pie Ranch welcomes casual visitors as well. The farm stand is situated just off of CA 1, about 11 miles south of Pescadero proper. With rustic wood construction, comfy chairs, twinkling lights, and friendly signs, it's an eminently quaint and welcoming stop on the scenic highway. Here you can buy pies, of course, made with fruits, nuts, and butter produced on the farm and baked in a commercial kitchen down the road at Companion Bakeshop (companionbakeshop.com) in Santa Cruz. The pies are as delicious as you'd expect, with a delicate whole-wheat crust and supremely fresh fillings. The farm stand also sells eggs, fruits, and veggies from the farm and a few souvenirs such as bumper stickers. Check the hours before visiting, however, because it's open only a few days a week and doesn't open until noon on weekdays.

13 SLIDE RANCH

2025 Shoreline Highway, Muir Beach, CA 94965; 415-381-6155, slideranch.org; open year-round. Detailed driving directions: slideranch.org/directions

WHAT THEY OFFER Camping, camps, event venue, hiking, kids' activities, picnicking, special events, training and internships

SITUATED ON 134 PICTURESQUE ACRES overlooking the bluffs of Muir Beach just half an hour north of San Francisco, Slide Ranch boasts a much more dramatic location than most working farms. Fortunately for all of us, a partnership with the Golden Gate National Recreation Area ensures that the grounds are open to the public for hiking, picnicking, and exploring all year long. And while casual visitors are politely asked to refrain from interacting with the goats, sheep, chickens, and ducks that call this spectacular location home, you can still explore the gardens and follow a hiking trail down to the beach, where rock-scrambling, wave-dodging, and tide-pooling adventures await.

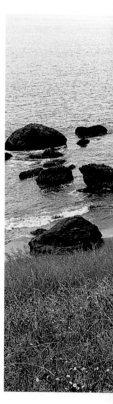

Slide Ranch was established in 1970 with the stated mission of connecting the Bay Area with "farm-based environmental education that focuses on the principles of sustainable agriculture and environmental stewardship." To that end, the organization offers camps, school field trips, and family programs year-round, teaching kids and adults about gardening, cooking, animal husbandry, and environmental stewardship. The nonprofit takes special interest in socioeconomically disadvantaged groups and those with physical and developmental disabilities. By offering financial aid to more than half of the students who participate in their programs every year, the folks at Slide Ranch ensure that their resources are available to people who don't typically get to participate in the farm-to-table movement.

Summer day camps on the ranch are offered to kids ages 5–13. Sessions last one week and are organized by age group, offering participants the opportunity to take care of farm animals, prepare meals with ingredients from the organic garden, and learn more about the natural world around them. Younger kids play games, enjoy story time, and do arts and crafts projects, while older kids more deeply explore the concept of environmental stewardship and learn about tide-pool ecology. Teenagers ages 14–18 are also invited to participate in a leadership role, assisting teachers-in-residence as junior camp counselors. The teachers-in-residence internship is offered to select emerging environmental educators, who not only lead the summer camp programs but also support the Slide Ranch staff in all aspects of maintaining a working farm throughout the year.

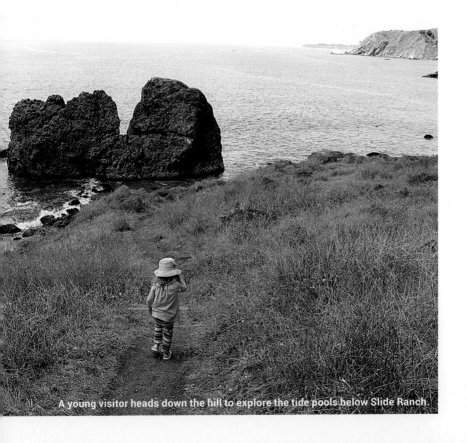

A young visitor heads down the hill to explore the tide pools below Slide Ranch.

While most of Slide Ranch's official programs are specifically for children and educators, seasonal activities such as family farm days and a harvest celebration give adults the opportunity to join their kids on the ranch. In addition to day-to-day farm activities such as collecting eggs, milking goats, and tending to the garden, participants also get to enjoy nature-inspired crafting projects and cooking workshops. Slide Ranch also occasionally offers families the opportunity to camp out on the property overnight.

Because Slide Ranch is a nonprofit dedicated to making its programs available to children of all socioeconomic levels, it relies heavily on the support of donors. A multitiered donation program details what exactly your money will support and offers incentives such as bumper stickers; note cards; and private garden parties, tours, and camp-outs. Visit the website to learn more about becoming involved with Slide Ranch and its devotion to farm-based environmental education.

TIPS Sunscreen and hats are a must if you plan to walk down to the beach, as the trail is very sunny. Be prepared to get wet while exploring the tide pools. This area can also cool down dramatically in cloudy weather and after dark, so bring a light jacket or sweater, as well.

14 TARA FIRMA FARMS

3796 I St., Petaluma, CA 94952; 707-765-1202, tarafirmafarms.com;
open year-round

WHAT THEY OFFER CSA, farm stand, special events, tours

LIKE MANY OF US, TARA AND CRAIG SMITH, the owners of Tara Firma
Farms, used to be regular nonfarming folk with city jobs and little connection to the food they ate. A copy of Michael Pollan's *The Omnivore's
Dilemma* changed all that: All at once, the couple took an intense interest in the food industry and, in particular, how flawed the industry was.
They read hundreds of books, watched documentaries, and sought
guidance from leaders in sustainable agriculture, such as Joel Salatin.
Then they decided to put their money where their mouths were, purchasing 290 acres of former dairy land just south of Petaluma.

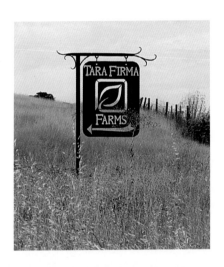

Today, Tara Firma Farms raises
pigs, chickens, turkeys, and
cows. All live and feed on pasture and are exposed to no
hormones or chemicals of any
kind. What exactly does it mean
to be pasture-raised? As tour
guide Dani explains, "It all starts
with grass." Tara Firma's herd
of cows is moved every day so
that they can continuously feed
on fresh, native grasses instead
of depleting the land of all veg-
etation. The soil is enriched with their manure, and after they've moved
on, a flock of chickens rotates through to do their business and enrich it
even further.

The pigs at Tara Firma have it pretty great as well. The farmers have
an arrangement with the local Costco and other local supermarkets
whereby they receive food that has passed its expiration date. This

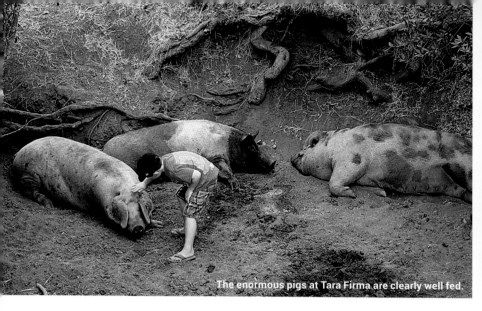

The enormous pigs at Tara Firma are clearly well fed.

means that their pigs get a never-ending feast of past-its-prime produce, breads, meats, and other items, which not only keeps all that waste out of the landfill but also keeps the pigs fat and healthy. Anything deemed unsuitable for even the pigs' consumption is tossed on the compost heap, and all the food containers are picked up and recycled. Tara Firma also has arrangements with local brewery Lagunitas and local cheese makers to collect the leftover grains and whey from the beer- and cheese-making processes, which they add to the pigs' feed as well. It doesn't get much greener than that.

Tara Firma raises chickens for both meat and eggs. Rather than maintain a hatchery on the premises, which involves too many staff to be cost effective, the farm orders its chicks from Iowa. Shipping poultry across the country may seem antithetical to the principles of local, sustainable agriculture, but Tara Firma has good reason: as it turns out, all of the eggs in West Coast hatcheries have been treated with a drop of antibiotics, which seeps through the permeable shell to the embryo within. That means that your so-called organic chicken may have been treated with antibiotics before it even had a chance to hatch (the organic label refers only to the animal's feed). For this reason, Tara Firma found a hatchery in Iowa that ships antibiotic-free chicks, which they then raise in their on-site brooder.

Tara Firma Farms has the classic farm feel that instantly evokes nostalgia, even for those with no personal history of farming. The original dairy structures still stand and now host nature camps for kids, barn dances, and other special events. The farm hosts free weekend tours for anyone interested in learning more about sustainable agricultural practices. And if you're lucky, resident grill master Tommy may even be serving up some freshly grilled sausages and hamburgers with a side of salad, all of it raised and produced on the farm, of course. This may be the most guilt-free meat you've ever eaten—and the most delicious.

Tara Firma sells its meat and eggs through a CSA home-delivery service throughout the Bay Area. In addition to the tours, seasonal events such as farm dinners, pumpkin-carving parties, and pig roasts are held throughout the year. Check the website to see what's coming up next.

TIPS You must live within the local delivery zone to subscribe to Tara Firma's CSA. But if you're in the area, you can always visit the on-site farm store, which is stocked with the same meat, eggs, organic produce, and other goodies. Check the website for hours. Also, street names can be a little confusing and redundant near the farm, so consider printing out a map to the location ahead of time as opposed to relying on GPS.

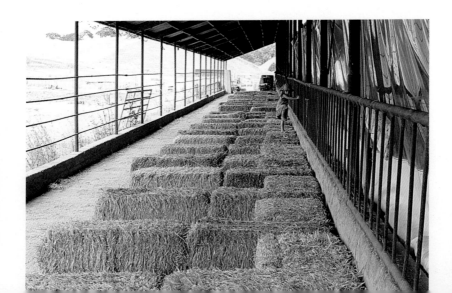

15 TOLUMA FARMS

5488 Middle Road, Tomales, CA 94971; 707-878-2142, tolumafarms.com. Open year-round; tours available by appointment.

WHAT THEY OFFER Lodging, tours

PRETTY MUCH ANY ROUTE YOU TAKE to Toluma Farms provides a breathtakingly beautiful journey. The rolling green hills of northwest Marin County are intermittently dotted with contented cows—long-haired ones, black ones, white and tan ones—and outlined with creeks and stands of madrone and eucalyptus trees, and the placid waters of Tomales Bay are just a few short miles away. In a region of California that isn't hurting in the least for scenery, the tiny town of Tomales still stands out. And Toluma Farms pretty much epitomizes the pastoral ideal. The working farm, dairy, and creamery offers 160 acres for its herd of 100 sheep and 180 goats to roam, meticulously employing pasture rotation to ensure that no section of land gets ravaged or over-stressed by the hungry animals.

Toluma's sheep and goats are milked once a day in the immaculate, state-of-the-art milking parlor near the front of the property. The milk is Grade A, meaning it can be sold and consumed directly in milk form as opposed to just being made into cheese and other products. That said, farmstead cheese is most definitely the name of the game here. At the Tomales Farmstead Creamery, located on the farm, artisanal-cheese makers craft soft-ripened goat cheese, aged hard goat cheese, an aged sheep-goat mix, and a three-day fresh farmer's cheese, all of which are named in the language of the Coast Miwok native people who used to live on this land. The cheeses are sold at the San Francisco Ferry Building, as well as some local farmers markets and Whole Foods locations.

A tour of Toluma Farms offers a comprehensive education in raising goats. You'll learn that female goats are typically bred at the age of 18 months (a few bucks reside on the farm for breeding), stop producing milk by the time they're 8 years old, and live to be 10–12 years old. Many of Toluma's elderly goats are sent to neighboring farms or offered to work for a local brush-clearing business. The goats are fed hay in the barn in the morning (Toluma Farms grows its own hay) and then allowed to graze on pasture for 6 hours a day. An intense system of pasture rotation—farm workers spend a great deal of time moving the temporary solar-powered electric fences from one field to another—ensures that there are always many acres of resting pasture, keeping the land healthy and fertile, not to mention picturesque as all get-out. About five different breeds of goats live on the farm, and these may be the friendliest farm animals you'll ever meet. They're alert, lively, and eager to nuzzle, clearly aware of just how lucky they are to be part of this sustainable, Animal Welfare Approved enterprise.

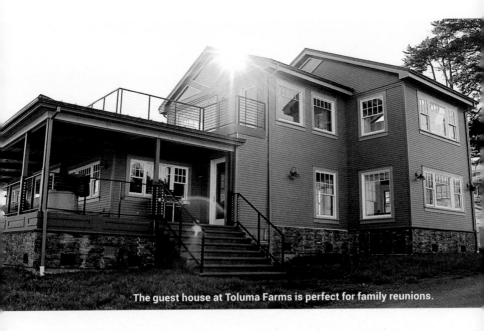

The guest house at Toluma Farms is perfect for family reunions.

Toluma Farms is located on the site of a former dairy and is now owned and operated by wife and husband Tamara Hicks and David Jablons, who purchased the property in 2003 and, after several years of intensive agricultural land restoration, started to raise livestock and make cheese in just the last few years. Tamara and David also rent out a large, modern country home on the property that's so gorgeous and beautifully appointed that it could be the setting of a show on the Food Network. The guesthouse sleeps 12–14 people and features a huge open kitchen, several bedrooms and a loft, bathrooms with claw-foot tubs, and a wraparound porch and upstairs deck offering stunning views of the surrounding pastures and rolling hills. Guests are welcome to tour the farm and get involved with some of the day-to-day chores.

Guided tours of Toluma Farms are offered to the public by appointment on the first Sunday of every month and offer visitors the chance to learn about the milking process, hike up to the pastures to meet the animals, and, of course, visit the creamery to taste the cheeses. Private tours for small groups and school field trips can also be arranged.

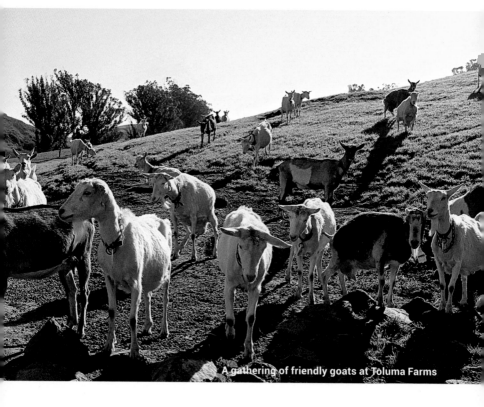
A gathering of friendly goats at Toluma Farms

ADDITIONAL FARMS IN THE AREA

Brentwood U-Pick Farms

Visit harvest4you.com to download a map of farms in the area.

Brentwood is home to a collection of pick-your-own farms popular with Bay Area families during the harvest season. Visitors can pick up a map of all area farm stands and farms and then go pick cherries, strawberries, boysenberries, nectarines, peaches, pears, plums, and more to their hearts' content. Most locations are open seasonally, and popular spots include Smith Family Farms, Pease Ranch, and Freitas Cherry Ranch.

City Slicker Farms

510-763-4241; visit cityslickerfarms.org for Community Market Farm locations.

Located in West Oakland, City Slicker Farms empowers low-income children and adults to grow, eat, and sell their own produce through several programs, including urban farming education, backyard gardening, and transforming empty lots into productive Community Market Farms. You can support their efforts by touring one of the Community Market Farms during open hours or by volunteering to help with a backyard garden build. Visit the website to learn about upcoming events and how to get involved.

Devil's Gulch Ranch

415-662-1099, devilsgulchranch.com; call for directions.

Located just a stone's throw from Cow Track Ranch (see page 32), Devil's Gulch Ranch is the site of DG Educational Services, a program whose stated mission is to "provide agriculture and nature educational programs to diverse communities, both locally and globally." To that end, the ranch hosts summer day camps and year-round programs to give kids the opportunity to experience rural life and become involved in the daily operations of a diversified animal and produce farm, all within the stunningly beautiful Golden Gate National Recreation Area.

Full Circle Farm

1055 Dunford Way, Sunnyvale, CA 94087; 408-475-2531, fullcirclesunnyvale.org

This community farm operates in partnership with the Santa Clara Unified School District to cultivate and maintain a local, sustainable food system in the area while also educating youth and adults alike about urban farming. Full Circle's produce is available at its farm stand and through a CSA membership. Volunteers are welcome in the farm's 1-acre Education Garden. Visit the website for farm stand and drop-in volunteer hours.

Green Gulch Farm Zen Center

1601 Shoreline Highway, Muir Beach, CA 94965; 415-383-3134, sfzc.org

The Green Gulch Farm Zen Center is just a few miles down the road from Slide Ranch (see page 52) and absolutely worth a visit if you're in Marin County. In addition to Zen meditation training, lectures, and retreats, the organization offers farm and garden work days and guest accommodations. The redwood groves of Mt. Tamalpais State Park are also nearby, offering world-class hiking and bicycle trails and spectacular views from the 2,571-foot peak.

Homeless Garden Project Farm

Delaware Avenue at Shaffer Road, Santa Cruz, CA 95060; 831-426-3609, homelessgardenproject.org

Just as the name implies, the Homeless Garden Project offers training, jobs, and support to the Santa Cruz homeless population. You can support their efforts by volunteering on the farm, in the kitchen, or at the retail store, as well as by signing up for the farm's CSA program. The organization also hosts regular fundraising farm dinners. Find dates and ticket info on the website.

McClelland's Dairy

6475 Bodega Ave., Petaluma, CA 94952; 707-664-0452, mcclellandsdairy.com

This family-run farm raises about 800 cows on 500 acres of pasture and hosts events throughout the year, including a pumpkin patch, school field trips, birthday parties, and traditional farm tours. Guests can enjoy organic grilled-cheese sandwiches and milk shakes at the food cart, and McClelland's also sells its artisan organic butter at stores throughout Marin, Napa, and Sonoma Counties.

McEvoy Ranch
5935 Red Hill Road, Petaluma, CA 94952; 866-617-6779, mcevoyranch.com

This sustainable olive ranch grows, harvests, mills, and bottles all of its own organic olive oils and has a wine tasting room. The ranch and tasting room are open by appointment only but do offer scheduled tours at certain times of the year. Visit the website to learn about upcoming tours and workshops or to book a private or corporate event at the ranch. McEvoy's products can also be sampled and purchased at its shop in the San Francisco Ferry Building Marketplace.

Open Field Farm
2245 Spring Hill Road, Petaluma, CA 94952; 707-775-4644, openfieldfarm.com

Open Field is a diversified farm dedicated to maintaining a balance between nature and cultivated land. The farmers here raise grass-fed beef, pastured eggs, chickens, and turkeys and grow a wide array of vegetables, flowers, and grains. Their products are available through a CSA subscription, and CSA members are invited to visit the farm a couple of times a week (in season) to choose what they want to take home and even harvest some of their own vegetables with the help of one of the farmers.

Swanton Berry Farm
25 Swanton Road, Davenport, CA 95017; 831-469-8804, swantonberryfarm.com

This charming little farm stand just off CA 1 between Pescadero and Santa Cruz has a pick-your-own-strawberry field and sells pies, strawberry lemonade and cider, and even hot soup (which can really hit the spot on this foggy, windswept coast). A sister property called Coastways Ranch also offers berry picking 10 minutes up the coast, at 640 CA 1 in Pescadero, but is open less often. Check the website for a picking schedule.

UC Santa Cruz Farm

1156 High St., Santa Cruz, CA 95064; 831-459-3240, casfs.ucsc.edu

UC Santa Cruz's Center for Agroecology & Sustainable Food Systems (CASFS) operates the small-scale, biodynamic Alan Chadwick Garden (named after the eccentric and renowned organic and biodynamic gardening pioneer), as well as a 30-acre farm, on the scenic UCSC campus. Both sites are certified organic and are internationally recognized horticultural and agricultural training and research grounds. The CASFS also operates Life Lab, a garden-based science and nutrition education nonprofit for pre-K through high school-age students. Visitors are welcome to visit both the farm and the garden daily, 8 a.m.–6 p.m.

Veggielution

Emma Prusch Farm Park, 647 S. King Road, San Jose, CA 95116; 888-343-6197, veggielution.org

This urban farm in the heart of Silicon Valley supplies fresh produce to the community—available every Saturday at its farm stand—and offers a discounted CSA membership to families in need. Regularly occurring programs include barn dances and children's activities in the youth garden. The organization welcomes volunteers and can also arrange group tours and community and corporate work days.

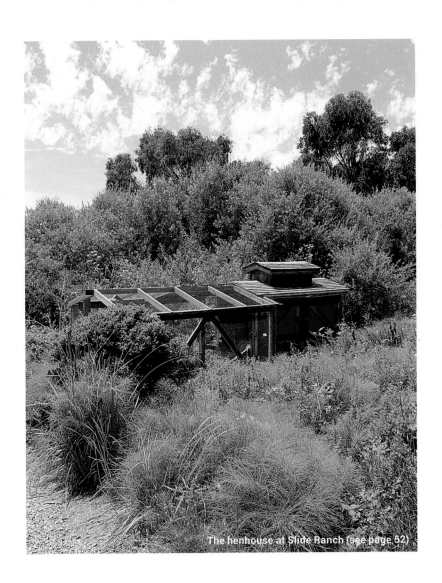

The henhouse at Slide Ranch (see page 52)

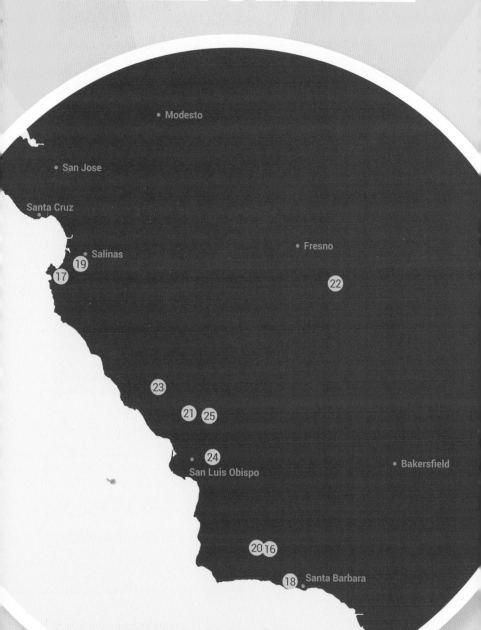

Central
CALIFORNIA

• Modesto

• San Jose

Santa Cruz

• Salinas
⑲
⑰

• Fresno

㉒

㉓

㉑ ㉕

㉔
San Luis Obispo

• Bakersfield

⑳⑯

⑱ • Santa Barbara

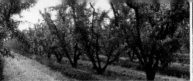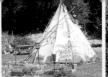

FARMS TO VISIT IN CENTRAL CALIFORNIA

16 CLAIRMONT FARMS

2480 Roblar Ave., Los Olivos, CA 93441; 805-688-7505, clairmontfarms.com;
open year-round

WHAT THEY OFFER Demonstrations, gift shop, picnicking

TUCKED AWAY ON A LITTLE HILL in the rustic wine-country town of
Los Olivos, Clairmont Farms is small but mighty. The 5-acre property is
home to Meryl Tanz and her son Sean Crowder, and—like much of the
land in the area—was formerly used to breed Thoroughbred horses. The
family started growing organic lavender here in 1998 and found a recep-
tive audience in both the local community and the many tourists who come
to Los Olivos to get the *Sideways* wine-tasting experience.

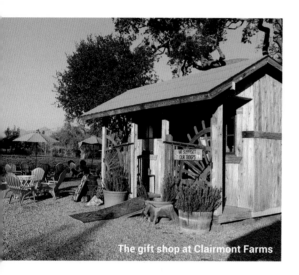

The gift shop at Clairmont Farms

Meryl and Sean started by planting 10,000 'Grosso' lavender plants,
which is a lavandin hybrid with an excep-
tionally high output of oil and buds. And as you
can imagine, their fields smell positively incredible when in bloom. Visitors are welcome to stroll
among the plants and picnic in the shade of the property's 300-year-old
oak trees. If you're there at the right time, you may even get a chance to
see the on-site copper distiller in action as it fills the air with an incredibly sweet and pure lavender essence like you've never experienced.

In addition to the strongly scented 'Grosso,' which is used for drying
into bundles and sachets and for bath and beauty products, Clairmont
grows 'Provence' lavender for culinary use. And if you get a chance to
sit down and chat with Meryl, she will share her many ideas for cooking

and preparing foods with Clairmont Farms' lavender pepper, lavender salt, and even just straight-up ground lavender buds—everything from lavender coffee and lavender-infused cocktails to lavender steak rubs and scrambled eggs. Meryl explains that the more mildly scented 'Provence' lavender works as a flavor enhancer in much the same way as saffron or salt, which makes it an extremely versatile herb.

Meryl and Sean rely on repeat business from both locals and out-of-towners, and their devotion to customer satisfaction and happiness is evident in their friendly, hospitable nature and generosity with their property. Naturally, the best time to visit Clairmont is in the spring, when the lavender fields are in their full blossoming glory. The scene is so picturesque that the farm is a popular venue for small weddings and photo shoots, but casual visitors are always welcome, as well. Children, in particular, get a kick out of frolicking through the purple fields. The family starts harvesting the fields in mid-June, but summer is also a lovely time to visit; you may find Meryl serving lavender cookies and lemonade to visitors as Sean demonstrates the distilling process. Really, if you're in the area any time of year, Clairmont Farms is worth a visit. Even when the fields are cut low and the weather is chilly, this is a friendly, bucolic, and welcoming place. And the charming gift shop set in the shade of an ancient oak tree is open year-round. Here you can purchase all manner of lavender seasonings, bath and beauty products, gift items, and, of course, dried lavender bundles and lavender essential oil straight from the fields.

TIP Watch out for bees! The fields are beautiful but buzzing when in bloom. Bees typically won't harm you if you don't bother them, but anyone with an allergy should beware when walking among the plants.

17 EARTHBOUND FARM STAND

7250 Carmel Valley Road, Carmel-by-the-Sea, CA 93923; 831-625-6219,
facebook.com/ebfarmstand; open year-round

WHAT THEY OFFER Classes and workshops, dining, farm stand,
gift shop, picnicking, special events

EARTHBOUND FARM ORGANIC IS A HUGE agricultural enterprise that
encompasses nearly 50,000 acres at multiple properties, but you
wouldn't know it from visiting their homey farm stand in Carmel
Valley. This sweet little Central Coast destination offers a glimpse into
the company's roots; founders Drew and Myra Goodman started
their original organic raspberry farm just down the road back in
1984. And while this throwback to a simpler time is quite a modest
operation by the company's current standards, calling this spot just a farm stand sells it short. With its
gorgeous surroundings, picnic area, market, café, and
interactive gardens, this is a destination in its own
right, not to mention a perfect excuse to visit the idyllic
Carmel Valley.

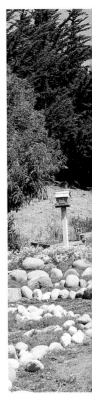

Although Earthbound grows a huge variety of produce, which is then sold through multiple retail outlets
throughout the country, the farm stand specializes in
herbs, berries, and flowers. The most interesting feature is an aromatherapy labyrinth, which incorporates
chamomile and other fragrant herbs and flowers as
a ground cover around the stones, adding a pleasing
sensory dimension to the contemplative practice of
walking its path. Beyond the labyrinth is a kids' garden
with a big, colorful tepee to explore. The property is
also home to flower fields and a raspberry patch, as
well as an herb garden and a kitchen garden, where
local chefs regularly host workshops. Additional special events take place throughout the year and include

herb- and flower-picking tours, "bug walks" for kids, lavender distilling demonstrations, pickling workshops, and seasonal happenings such as pumpkin-carving and holiday wreath-making days. Some events are free and open to drop-in visitors, while others charge a fee and require reservations. The best way to stay on top of upcoming events is to visit the farm stand's Facebook page.

Casual visitors are always welcome to drop by, as well, to walk through the gardens and enjoy a picnic on the grounds. Earthbound's on-site café serves an all-certified-organic menu of salads, sandwiches, soups, pizzas, juices, and smoothies, and the adjoining market sells a carefully curated selection of organic snacks, baked goods, fresh meat and dairy items, meals to go, and, of course, locally grown fruits and vegetables. Visitors are welcome to enjoy their food in the covered picnic pavilion or to bring a blanket and stretch out on the lawn.

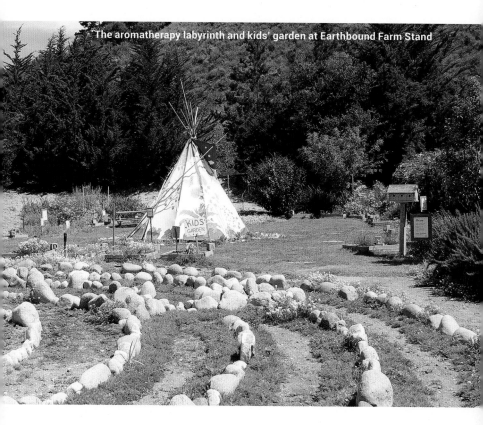

The aromatherapy labyrinth and kids' garden at Earthbound Farm Stand

The Earthbound Farm Stand is just a few miles inland from the wealthy coastal community of Carmel-by-the-Sea and only about 15 minutes from Monterey, so it should certainly be a planned stop on any trip to the peninsula. And Carmel Valley itself is a gorgeous, typically sunny destination, with plenty of opportunities for golfing and wine tasting. The nearby Carmel Valley Ranch is a family-friendly resort that incorporates the region's agricultural heritage into the hospitality experience with lavender fields, vineyards, a big organic garden, and beekeeping classes; it's a great place to stay if you're looking to splurge on accommodations in the area (see sidebar).

TIP Because the Earthbound Farm Stand has its own café and market, visitors are respectfully asked to purchase their meals on-site rather than bring their own food to picnic on the property.

NEARBY ATTRACTION Carmel Valley Ranch

Sprawling and scenic, Carmel Valley Ranch is in many ways your typical upscale golf resort, featuring multiple pools and hot tubs, a renowned restaurant, and its own private vineyard. But what sets this destination apart is its embrace of agritourism. Guests are welcome to wander through acres of lavender fields (most magnificent in late spring and early summer, but watch out for bees) and to visit the resort's beautiful culinary garden. Organic farmer extraordinaire Mark Marino (who, as it happens, also helped build and develop the Earthbound Farm Stand) is typically around on Saturday mornings and always happy to chat with guests about gardening. Mark designed the garden with both beauty and functionality in mind—tall flowers and vines like sunflowers, hollyhock, and hops add color, height, and texture, while most of the vegetable beds are devoted to heirloom varieties requested by the resort's executive chef, Tim Wood. The garden is also home to a chicken coop; an apiary, where guests can sign up for beekeeping classes; and even a salt house, where Monterey Bay Salt Co. dries sea salt from deep in the bay's pristine waters. Carmel Valley Ranch's dedication to the area's agricultural heritage is apparent, and its educational food production offerings make it stand out from Carmel's other high-end hotels and resorts.

1 Old Ranch Road, Carmel-by-the-Sea, CA 93923; 855-OUR-RANCH, carmelvalleyranch.com

18 FAIRVIEW GARDENS

598 N. Fairview Ave., Goleta, CA 93117; 805-967-7369, fairviewgardens.org; open year-round

WHAT THEY OFFER Apprenticeships, camps, classes and workshops, farm stand, tours

AS YOU DRIVE PAST THE MINI-MALLS and fast-food restaurants lining Fairview Avenue on your way to Fairview Gardens, it may be hard to believe that you're approaching what may be the oldest organic farm in Southern California. Founded back in 1895, this fertile 12.5 acres has managed to survive despite the commercial and residential development that has encroached on all sides. This is thanks to an agricultural conservation easement, which will ensure that the nonprofit farm will continue to operate, educate, and serve the growing suburban community that surrounds it for many years to come.

The land was owned by the Chapman family in the 1970s, and it was patriarch Roger Chapman's vision to maintain the organic family farm as an educational facility for the community. When Roger passed away in 1994, longtime Farm Manager Roger Ableman formed a nonprofit organization to buy the farm and place it in trust with the Land Trust for Santa Barbara County. The official name of the nonprofit that now operates the farm is the Center for Urban Agriculture, and it's the organization's duty to keep Fairview Gardens as a working organic farm with an emphasis on community education.

The diversified urban farm is located on the former site of a Chumash settlement where the topsoil is incredibly rich, making it perfect for cultivation. In the 19th and early 20th centuries, the Goleta Valley became an agricultural mecca, particularly for citrus groves. Development wasn't far behind, though, and the Santa Barbara Airport and University of California, Santa Barbara, moved into the area in the 1940s and '50s, followed soon thereafter by miles and miles of housing tracts. All of this development puts Fairview Gardens in the perfect position to make farming convenient and accessible to a great number of people who would normally have no exposure to agriculture.

In addition to serving hundreds of local families through its CSA, farmers markets, and farm stand, Fairview offers after-school classes and summer camps for kids, as well as tours, workshops, and apprenticeships for adults. The huge array of learning opportunities available to the public is a sign of how invested the Center for Urban Agriculture is in the surrounding community, and the concept of mentorship is huge here. Fairview's staff members and apprentices are devoted to fostering a love of nature and connection to the land in the children who participate in their year-round programs. With abundant avocado and mulberry trees to climb, animals to care for, and a dedicated, highly interactive children's garden, this place is absolute heaven for kids. Adults, too, can learn at the farm through homesteading classes on topics such as raising backyard chickens, baking bread, or building an outdoor cob oven.

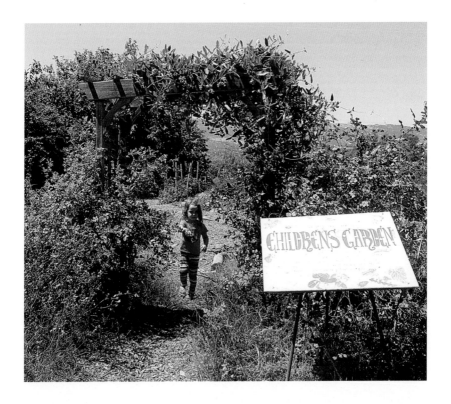

Fairview Gardens is open to casual visitors, as well. The bright and cheery farm stand is located right on the street, offering fresh-picked produce from its own fields, as well as from a handful of other local growers. Here you can also purchase coffee, popcorn, honey, preserves, nuts, and other goodies. You can also pick up a map and take a self-guided tour of the farm (technically free, although cash donations are welcomed). The walking tour gives visitors an idea of the impressive diversity of this small working farm, which grows a broad array of fruit and vegetable crops throughout SoCal's long growing season and is home to goats and chickens. Docent-led tours are also available to schools and other groups who want to take a more in-depth look at Fairview Gardens' practices and mission and can be arranged through the website.

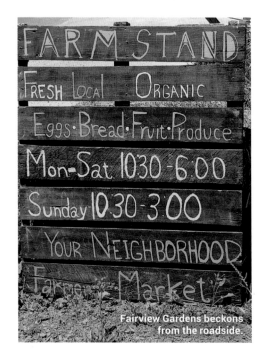

Fairview Gardens beckons from the roadside.

19 THE FARM IN SALINAS

7 Foster Road, Salinas, CA 93902; 831-455-2575, thefarm-salinasvalley.com; open spring, summer, and fall

WHAT THEY OFFER CSA, farm stand, kids' activities, seasonal events, tours

THE FIRST THING YOU'LL NOTICE AS YOU APPROACH The Farm in Salinas, which is a few miles off US 101 on CA 68, is the giant plywood sculptures by artist John Cerney. These outsize tributes to the hard-working farmers of the Salinas Valley realistically depict the various labors of farming, from checking the soil and planting to harvesting and packing, in sun-drenched living color. At up to 18 feet tall, they can be a little jarring at first sight but are undeniably beautiful, and serve as effective and unusual billboards for The Farm. If you drive I-5 through the heart of California's Central Valley, you may come across Cerney's artwork at other farms, as well. They serve as a slightly surreal, and entirely welcome, visual stimulus on what can be a monotonous journey.

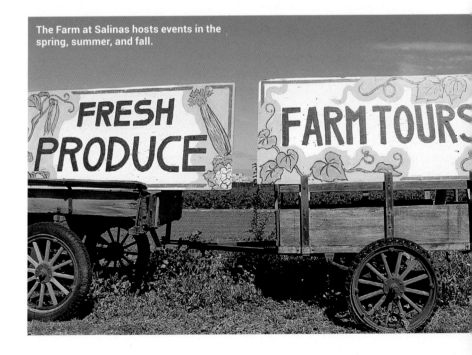

The Farm at Salinas hosts events in the spring, summer, and fall.

Salinas is only about 10 miles inland and less than 20 miles from Monterey but feels very much like a Central Valley farming town. The Salinas Valley is often referred to as "the salad bowl of the world" because such an abundance of lettuce crops are grown here. And while agriculture is undeniably the main endeavor around these parts, Salinas' Oldtown area offers plenty of modern comforts housed behind charming brick storefronts, such as cafés, boutiques, breweries, and Pilates studios. For literature buffs, the National Steinbeck Center (the author was born here; see sidebar) is absolutely worth a visit.

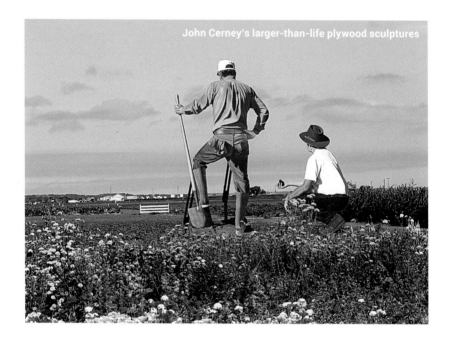
John Cerney's larger-than-life plywood sculptures

Throughout the growing season The Farm grows about 30 different crops, including strawberries, lettuces, corn, and tomatoes—mostly organic—which are available through a CSA subscription and at the on-site produce stand. In addition to marketing its fruits and vegetables, The Farm is dedicated to educating the public about agriculture through farm tours. Group tours last about an hour and include a tractor ride and an overview of farming in the Salinas Valley; custom tours can also be arranged. These tours can last 1, 2, or 3 hours and give participants the chance to be more involved in the farming process, from working with machinery to thinning crops to packing produce boxes.

The Farm also offers school field trips and special learning events aimed at families, such as Honey Day and Worm Day, as well as good old-fashioned farm fun, such as hayrides, watermelon-eating contests, and pumpkin tosses, depending on the season. If you aren't in town for one of these scheduled events and haven't scheduled a tour, but happen to be passing through the area Monday–Saturday, you can always stop by the farm stand for fresh produce. Fresh-baked fruit pies are sold in the farm shop on Fridays. The farm is generally closed Christmas–April for the winter season but is open on certain dates during this period to sell pies. Be sure to check the website before visiting to make sure the farm is open to the public and to find out about upcoming events.

NEARBY ATTRACTION National Steinbeck Center

Located in the heart of Oldtown Salinas, the National Steinbeck Center celebrates the literature and legacy of John Steinbeck by offering exhibits and events that explore history, art, literature, and agriculture in the heart of Steinbeck country.

1 Main St., Salinas, CA 93901; 831-775-4721, steinbeck.org

GLOBAL GARDENS

2450 Alamo Pintado Road, Solvang, CA 93463 (it's actually in Los Olivos); 800-307-0447, globalgardensonline.com; open year-round, Friday–Sunday

WHAT THEY OFFER Classes and workshops, gift shop, tasting

IN 1998, THEODORA STEPHAN LEFT HER CAREER as a graphic designer and started growing Italian, Greek, and Spanish olive tree varietals on her 3 acres in Los Olivos. She was inspired by her Greek heritage and her love of cooking to start making her own gourmet extra-virgin olive oils, and Global Gardens was born.

Theo found success in pressing, bottling, and selling her oils, as well as homemade natural fruit vinegars, and even expanded her business to operate a thriving café for a period of time. But she has now reinvented her business to incorporate a strong educational component by converting her land into a demonstration garden dubbed the Fast Food Farm. Theo has always happily advised her customers on the tastiest uses for each of her olive oil varietals and balsamic vinegars, not to mention their considerable health benefits. And now she also offers permaculture, pruning and canning workshops, and other instructional support for people who, like her, want to achieve sustainable self-sufficiency in their own backyards. A mother of two young adult daughters, Theo is particularly homed in on millennials. As she puts it, "We baby boomers spent a lot of time and money living the good life." As far as she's concerned, it's now her generation's responsibility to inspire and support young people in their attempt to shift the world toward sustainable agricultural practices.

Theo may have taken on a weighty mission, but that doesn't mean her demo garden and farm stand aren't fun to visit. Open Friday, Saturday, and Sunday or by appointment, the tasting room and boutique is open, airy, and inviting; filled with light; and surrounded by silvery olive trees. Here you can meet Theo and sample Global Gardens' many varieties of organic, first-cold-press, extra-virgin olive oils, as well as her delicious balsamic vinegars made with fruits and herbs, many of which she grew herself. One of Theo's niftiest creations is a custom tasting kit. Modeled on a painter's palette, the kit holds seven oils and five vinegars. Theo can walk you through the tasting, explaining how each oil's distinctive flavor is determined by the olive varietal, the terroir (the landscape where the trees were grown), and how ripe the olives were when pressed. She'll also gladly share recipes and ideas for how to prepare meals and cook with each of the oils and vinegars.

The store also sells some of Theo's homemade pantry items, such as spiced nuts, jars of olives and mustard, and custom seasoning blends, and is a popular stop for wine tours looking to break up a day of drinking with some delicious, locally made snacks. For true olive oil lovers and gourmet cooks, Global Gardens also offers several mail-order subscription-club options.

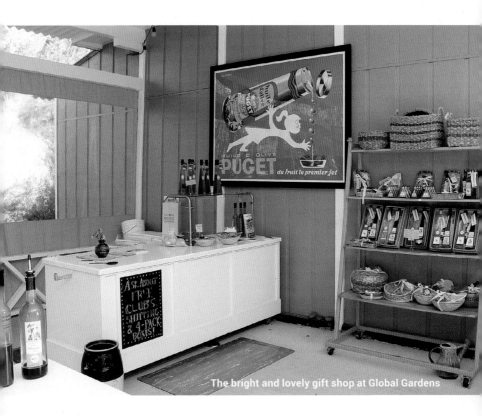

The bright and lovely gift shop at Global Gardens

21 KILER RIDGE

1111 Kiler Canyon Road, Paso Robles, CA 93446; 805-400-1439, kilerridge.com; open year-round

WHAT THEY OFFER Picnicking, tasting, tours

KILER RIDGE IS LOCATED IN THE HEART of the Central Coast's wine country, amid Paso Robles's many tasting rooms and vineyards. However, this farm exults the olive far above the grape, producing some of the finest Tuscan-style olive oils you'll find outside of Italy.

To reach the milling facility and tasting room, you'll follow a winding road to the top of a hill, and then enter through Kiler Ridge's massive gates. Atop the hill, views of the surrounding olive tree orchards and Paso Robles's farms and vineyards abound. In the sustainably designed tasting and milling facility, one of Kiler Ridge's associates will offer an education in olive oil, followed by samples of several of the farm's

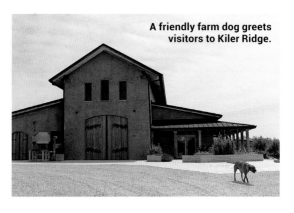

A friendly farm dog greets visitors to Kiler Ridge.

varietals. Trust us: You will taste the difference between these extraordinarily fresh, cold-pressed oils and the crud you've been buying at the grocery store all these years. In fact, you'll probably be more than a little chagrined to discover that much of the imported olive oil you've been buying and cooking with is actually rancid due to the lack of stringent labeling rules for oil sold in the United States (and the expensive testing procedure required to determine if mass-produced oil has gone rancid before it's distributed to grocery stores). This isn't to say that rancid oil smells or tastes especially bad to the average American palate—indeed, it's what many of us have become accustomed to. However, once one of Kiler Ridge's associates walks you through the process of determining the good from the bad, you'll walk away with a more refined palate and a vow never to consume that nasty old stuff again.

The tasting begins with a sample of a popular name-brand, midpriced "extra virgin" olive oil widely available in the supermarket. Chances are, it will taste just as it should to you at first. Next comes a palate cleanser of fresh sliced apples, followed by a sampling of several of Kiler Ridge's offerings. The process is eye-opening and delicious; your guide will instruct you on how to smell, taste, and feel on your tongue the difference between fresh olive oil and that which has gone bad and been chemically processed, not to mention the striking differences in flavor between Kiler's own varieties (such as the newly pressed *olio nuovo*, which is peppery, vibrant, nutty, and best suited for drizzling over bread, veggies, and cooked meats) and one of its everyday varieties, which are typically mellower in flavor and used for cooking. While you're there, treat yourself to an olive oil and ice cream tasting—you'll never want to eat vanilla without olive oil and sea salt again.

Kiler Ridge refers to its tasting room and production facility as the farm's *frantoio*, or "olive mill" in Italian. The beautiful building is insulated with straw bales and is solar-powered, making it incredibly energy efficient. In addition to visiting the tasting room, you have the option of taking a 90-minute olive oil production tour or a 30-minute walking tour of the orchard. Tours and tastings are offered several days a week; find a full schedule on the Kiler Ridge website.

TIPS Bring a picnic lunch or simply a loaf of fresh bread to enjoy with the olive oil you will inevitably feel inspired to purchase after your tasting. Kiler Ridge encourages visitors to linger on its lovely, rustically furnished patio overlooking the orchards and Paso Robles countryside.

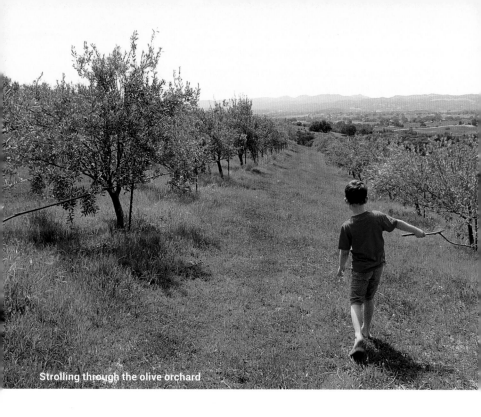

Strolling through the olive orchard

NEARBY ATTRACTION Firestone Walker Brewing Co.

Paso Robles may be known as wine country, but if you're in the mood for something sudsier and a hearty meal, head over to the Firestone Walker Brewing Co. and Taproom Restaurant, just a few miles away from Kiler Ridge on the other side of US 101. The popular Central Coast brewing company has a loyal following (even outside of the 805 area code), and you can sample more than a dozen of their brews here, as well as take a complimentary tour of the brewery.

1400 Ramada Drive, Paso Robles, CA 93446; 805-225-5911, firestonebeer.com

22 NAYLOR'S ORGANIC FAMILY FARM

38918 Road 64, Dinuba, CA 93618; 559-591-6051, naylorsorganicfarmstay.com. Farm-stay availability varies by season but is typically offered Wednesday–Saturday nights spring–fall. U-pick is offered May–September.

WHAT THEY OFFER Lodging, tours, U-pick

THERE'S AN AWFUL LOT TO LIKE ABOUT STAYING at Naylor's Organic Family Farm, but the main draw is undoubtedly the Naylors themselves. Warm, welcoming, and convivial as can be, they quickly make you feel like you're staying with family or close friends. Mike is gregarious—full of stories and bons mots—while Nori comes off as patient, maternal, and placid, but don't be fooled; she has a great sense of humor and some stories to tell, as well. The former high school sweethearts have grand-kids of their own now and are as welcoming toward children as adults. Kids are sure to love Penny the farm dog—the sweet Vizsla is gentle and tolerant toward little ones. (Be warned: She might greet you with a cottontail in her mouth. That's farm life.)

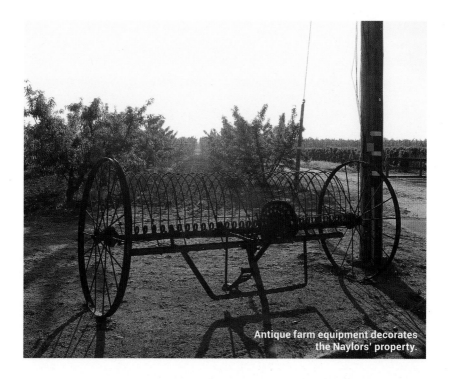

Antique farm equipment decorates the Naylors' property.

The Forestiere Underground Gardens are just over a half an hour north of Dinuba and are a marvel of human ingenuity and hard work that truly must be seen to be believed. Located on busy West Shaw Avenue in Fresno, this attraction doesn't look like much from the street. But don't let that stop you from signing up for a tour; once you head underground with your guide, you will be amazed at what Sicilian immigrant Baldassare Forestiere built here between 1906 and 1946.

Baldassare, whose work history included digging subway tunnels in Boston, originally bought the land to plant orchards but was dismayed to hit hardpan (which has the consistency of cement) not far below the topsoil. This major agricultural snag, combined with a desire to escape the summer heat of the Central Valley, inspired Forestiere to dig out an entire subterranean home for himself. He discovered good soil below the hardpan, so he dug his way through and used the hardpan, along with mortar and cement, to reinforce the walls, arches, and ceilings of his underground retreat. A horticulturist at heart, Baldassare even planted many varieties of fruit trees underground, exposing the plants to the sun via skylights, and many of those trees still thrive and produce fruit today. Over the years, he expanded his network of subterranean rooms, tunnels, grottoes, and gardens to total 10 acres, with dreams of operating a subterranean resort for other locals in search of hot-weather relief.

Sadly, a significant portion of Baldassare's incredible creation was demolished after he died with the construction of I-99. But what remains is nonetheless remarkable and a must-see destination for anyone traveling through the Fresno area. Tours are offered several days a week and last about an hour.

5021 W. Shaw Ave., Fresno, CA 93722; 559-271-0734,
undergroundgardens.com

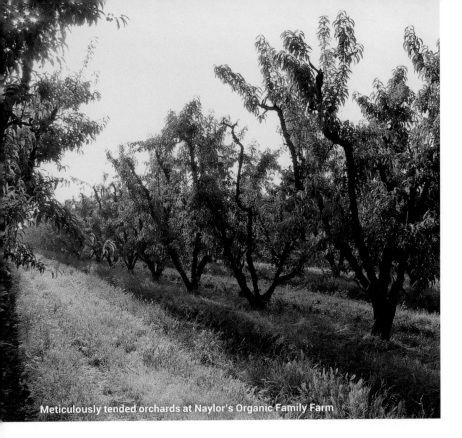
Meticulously tended orchards at Naylor's Organic Family Farm

Mike Naylor is a third-generation farmer, and the land on which he grows his peaches and nectarines has been in his family since 1963. He started farming himself in 1979, and the whole operation went completely organic in 1984, so the Naylor family farmers are pioneers in that regard. To say that farming is in Mike's blood is an understatement; this man knows his property inside and out, and his affection for both the land and the fruit it produces is evident. Naylor's Organic produces about 25 varieties of stone fruit—many are rare varieties developed by a since-retired heritage grower—on 65 acres of land. (The property totals 95 acres, but California's ongoing drought has caused Mike to fallow some of his fields.) Farm-stay guests are welcome to tour the farm with Mike, who will gladly share the ins and outs of organic farming in the Central Valley. While the farm employs about 20 workers, Mike is incredibly hands-on and can explain the details of irrigation, crop thinning, rototilling, harvesting, and any other topic you may be curious about.

If you visit in the summer, you'll find him busy at work in the orchards. Unlike most stone-fruit growers, Naylor still packs the fruit in the fields at peak ripeness, resulting in immensely sweet, flavorful fruit that has been meticulously handled to prevent bruising.

The Naylors like to think of their home as a relaxing way station for travelers through the Central Valley and, to that end, don't have the two-night minimum that many farm stays require. But staying here is such a pleasure that many visitors book for a couple of nights or even a full week. Two bedrooms are available in the house, each with a private bathroom, refrigerator, and separate entrance. The accommodations are comfortable, well appointed, and spotless—Nori will warn you that life on the farm includes bugs and thoughtfully provides a handheld vacuum for sucking up wayward insects, but you probably won't need it. Guests are in for a treat at breakfast time, when Nori cooks up a feast that may include sausages, scrambled eggs, hash browns, fresh fruit, blackberry muffins, and fresh-squeezed orange juice. And once you've eaten a hearty breakfast and toured the farm, the Naylor residence makes an excellent jumping-off point for hiking the trails and marveling at the giant sequoias of Kings Canyon and Sequoia National Parks, which are about an hour or so away.

If you are just passing through the area and don't have time to spend the night, visit Naylor's to pick your own blackberries, peaches, and nectarines. Dedicated U-pick orchards and fields on the farm offer their own unique varieties for road trippers eager to sample the local flavor. Mike and Nori educate visitors on how to tell when the fruit is ready to be picked, and they offer tasting, as well. Harvest season typically runs mid-May–September, but call ahead to confirm that the fruit is ready to be picked.

23 RANCHO DOS AMANTES

222 Wendy Way, Bradley, CA 93426; 805-472-2878, ranchodosamantes.com; open year-round. Detailed driving directions: ranchodosamantes.com/directions

WHAT THEY OFFER Classes and workshops, event venue, lodging, tours (available to farm stay guests)

TAMERA CLIFFORD AND HER FAMILY have created the perfect amalgam of rustic farm stay and cushy bed-and-breakfast on their 49-acre ranch outside of Paso Robles. Visitors travel 25 miles of scenic winding road after exiting US 101 to reach the property and, once there, will find no TVs or Wi-Fi to distract from the feeling of total country escape.

It was that sense of escape that drew Tamera and her husband, Jeff, to this beautiful plot of land in the first place. Like many city-folk-turned-farmers, Tamera and Jeff started with just a modest edible garden, but their appreciation for the lifestyle led them to expand into livestock, with a flock of chickens, a small herd of Nubian goats, and even a llama. The gardens have grown, as well, and Rancho Dos Amantes now includes two

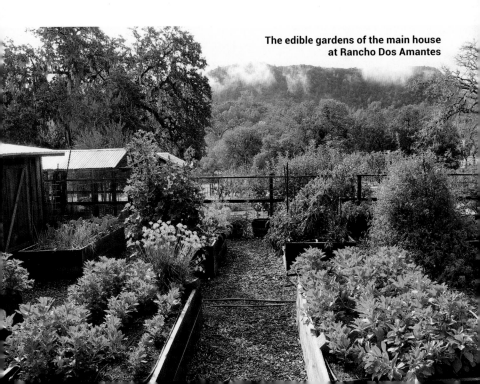

The edible gardens of the main house at Rancho Dos Amantes

expansive raised vegetable gardens—one for the main house and one for guests to harvest from—as well as olive, apple, and stone-fruit orchards.

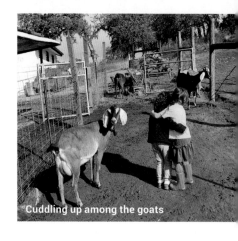
Cuddling up among the goats

With only a few rooms available, Rancho Dos Amantes is a fairly intimate B&B and is especially well suited for family reunions, wedding parties, or two or three families traveling together, although it makes a lovely retreat for couples, as well. Lodging options include two standalone casitas and a private apartment located above the Red Barn Kitchen, the fully equipped commercial kitchen and dining area, which is available to all guests and serves as the de facto gathering place on the property. All guest quarters are comfortable, immaculate, and decorated in tasteful country-chic style, and the grounds include a lush green lawn for stargazing, cartwheeling, croquet, and fire pits (marshmallows, cozy blankets, wood, and kindling are provided) looking out over the ranch's hay fields and the rolling hills in the distance.

Every morning, guests get to enjoy a farm-style Continental breakfast in the Red Barn Kitchen, which will likely include fruit, yogurt, granola, and one or more options of delectable, freshly baked breads. Afterward, Tamera is happy to take guests up to the property of the main house to meet Scarlet the llama, pet the friendly goats, and gather eggs from the chickens. *Note:* The main farm is just a short distance uphill—easily walkable, but kids will no doubt enjoy a ride with Tamera on the Kawasaki Mule UTV.

Located near the border between Monterey and San Luis Obispo Counties, Rancho Dos Amantes makes a solid home base for exploring the Central Coast. The charming towns of Arroyo Grande, Cayucos, and Morro Bay are all just a little over an hour's drive away and well worth exploring. If you're up for adventure, go zip-lining at Margarita

Adventures in Santa Margarita (see page 100) or tackle the ropes courses at Vista Lago Adventure Park in the Lopez Lake Recreation Area (vistalagoadventurepark.com). In addition to the farm stay, Tamera offers cooking classes and hands-on ranch dinners at the Red Barn Kitchen and can also host weddings or other special events on the property.

> **TIP** Be sure to designate a driver if you plan to hit up the many wineries in the area—those winding country roads are no joke. Better yet, just bring a bottle back to your casita and enjoy it from the scenic comfort of a rocking chair on your private patio.

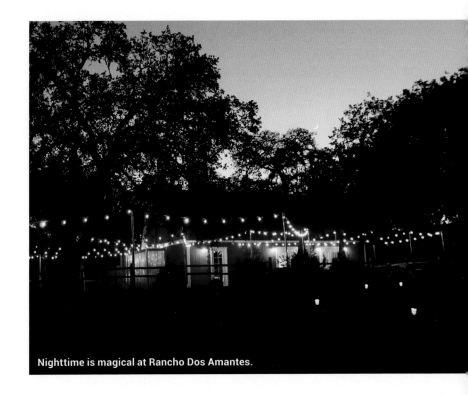

Nighttime is magical at Rancho Dos Amantes.

RINCONADA DAIRY

4680 W. Pozo Road, Santa Margarita, CA 93453; 805-438-5667 rinconadadairy.com; open year-round

WHAT THEY OFFER Hiking, lodging, tours (all activities available to farm-stay guests only)

AT THIS 92-ACRE RANCH IN SAN LUIS OBISPO COUNTY, farm owners Christine and Jim Maguire open their home to guests, whom they fortify with delicious farm-fresh breakfasts and gladly instruct in the ways of milking, tending to livestock, and organic gardening. The ranch is home to dozens of pigs, sheep, and goats; the latter two provide the milk to make the dairy's renowned cheeses, available at some SoCal farmers markets and high-end cheese stores. What's more, Christine and Jim just about perfectly manifest the typical urban or suburban preconception of what farmers should be: practical, hardworking, and dedicated to common-sense good eating and living. Christine has the demeanor of a favorite aunt—all wry humor

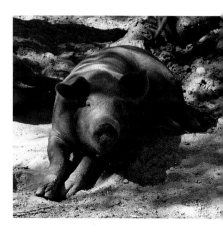

and no-nonsense straightforwardness—while Jim is soft-spoken and good-natured, just as patient with a woefully agriculturally ignorant adult as he is with a boisterous kid.

Guests at Rinconada have two lodging options. The guest wing of the main house can accommodate two adults in the beautifully decorated bedroom and offers access to a private bathroom and pleasant reading nook (with plenty of good books provided). Staying in the main house includes the perk of being served a fully prepared breakfast every morning in the type of farmhouse kitchen you'd expect to see in a Nora Ephron movie. The hearty items offered may include buttery apple cake, scrambled eggs straight from the henhouse, freshly picked berries with goat's milk yogurt, or exquisite homemade sausage patties courtesy of one of the farm's former porcine residents.

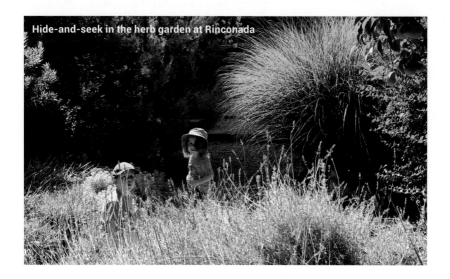
Hide-and-seek in the herb garden at Rinconada

If you have more people in your group or simply want a little more independence, you can stay in the well-appointed and comfortable private apartment built into the barn. With a fully equipped kitchen, bedroom, and sofa bed in the front room, the apartment can accommodate up to four people. Staying here, you'll forgo the fully prepared gourmet breakfast but will find your kitchen stocked with eggs, goat's milk and yogurt, bacon and sausage, and fresh-baked bread so you can prepare meals at your leisure.

TIPS The Rinconada ranch is a great area to hike and explore, but rattlesnakes and poison oak are real risks. Plan to wear long pants and high-top shoes if you plan to do any off-the-beaten-path adventuring. Mornings can be quite chilly, even in the spring, so bring warm clothes if you plan to rise for the morning farm rounds.

Jim and Christine are happy either to show guests around the farm or to simply go about their own business, so a stay at Rinconada is whatever you choose to make of it. If your idea of the perfect getaway involves maneuvering 75-pound bales of hay and milking goats, wake up early (or be around at 5 p.m.) and ride around in a John Deere Gator mini-tractor with Jim and a couple of farm dogs during the morning and evening milking and feeding rounds. Alternatively, you can approach farm life at a more leisurely pace by waking up whenever you want, gathering your own fresh produce from the garden for meals, and simply wandering around the ranch to say hello to the farm animals and hike up rocky hillsides in search of the American Indian grinding holes that were once used to grind acorns into flour. The farm's location is remote enough to provide a peaceful sense of true rural solitude, but because the 101 freeway is only about 15–20 minutes away, it's a relatively short and easy jaunt to Avila Beach, San Luis Obispo, and Paso Robles, making this a great jumping-off point to explore the Central Coast.

NEARBY ATTRACTION The Range

Rustic yet upscale, with a welcoming patio and an excellent farm-fresh menu with plenty of delectable meat options as well, The Range is a destination unto itself in San Luis Obispo County and is only about a 15-minute drive from Rinconada Dairy. You'll likely find Rinconada's cheeses featured in some of the dishes, along with produce from local farms. Be sure to bring cash— credit cards aren't accepted. Also note that the restaurant is closed Sunday and Monday.

22317 El Camino Real, Santa Margarita, CA 93453; 805-438-4500 (no website)

25 **WINDROSE FARM**

5750 El Pharo Drive, Paso Robles, CA 93446; 805-239-3757, windrosefarm.org.
Open year-round, Tuesday–Saturday; call ahead to book a farm tour. Detailed
driving directions: windrosefarm.org/about-us/directions.

WHAT THEY OFFER Camping, classes and workshops, farm stand,
lodging, special events, tours

WINDROSE FARM SUPPLIES ITS ORGANIC PRODUCE to some of Los
Angeles's finest restaurants and is a mainstay at the big Santa Monica
and Hollywood farmers markets, favorites of discerning local chefs.
Fortunately, when you spend time at this small family farm outside
of Paso Robles, the big city and all of the glamour and pretense of
its dining scene couldn't seem farther away. To get to Windrose,
you must exit the highway and travel several miles of country roads,
passing rustic wineries, olive groves, horse ranches, and homesteads
before eventually arriving at the long dirt road that leads to the farm.
By the time you arrive, you'll have the distinct sensation that you've
"gotten away from it all."

The beautiful 50-acre property is overseen by Barbara and Bill Spen-
cer, a former studio musician and real estate agent, respectively, who
caught the organic farming bug back in the early 1990s and quickly
developed an affinity for sustainable practices such as composting and
cover-cropping, as well as for growing heirloom varieties of tomatoes,
potatoes, apples, and other fruits and vegetables. The Spencers are
now taking things even further as they pursue biodynamic standards.
To that end, they make all of their own fertilizer blends and take advantage of the many horse ranches in the area to build their compost.

Much of the Windrose land is an uncultivated natural habitat for wildlife, and only a couple of dozen acres are devoted to vegetable fields,
orchards, and sheep pasture. Bill and Barbara are fortunate in that all
of that surrounding wild land means no potential contamination from
conventional farming operations. What's more, the farm's location in
the often shaded valley translates into more "chill hours" for its fruit
trees, allowing the Spencers to grow many specialty apple varieties

that won't grow anywhere else in the area. The icing on the cake? Windrose Farm is located atop a natural aquifer, and its two wells haven't yet run dry, despite the multiyear drought. The appeal of this piece of land is abundantly clear, and it comes as no surprise that the boomerang-shaped valley, with its fertile soil, natural water supply, and plentiful shade trees, was part of an ancient American Indian migration route.

The Spencers open Windrose to the public Tuesday–Saturday, when visitors are welcome to take a self-guided tour of the farm and visit the charming farm stand. In addition to seasonal fruits and vegetables, the on-site shop sells olive oil and cheeses from nearby farms (including Rinconada Dairy, page 92), along with soaps, gardening books, and other gift items. And on a hot summer day, nothing tastes better than one of the gourmet ice pops from the freezer. Guided tours of the farm are also offered on Saturdays for $10 per person, and seasonal camping is available in the orchard for $20 per night. If you'd like to stay on the property but don't have camping gear, book a farm stay in the Treehouse Trailer, so named because it's located next to a gorgeous 100-year-old oak tree. Windrose also hosts special events throughout the year, including farm dinners, tomato tasting, and gardening workshops.

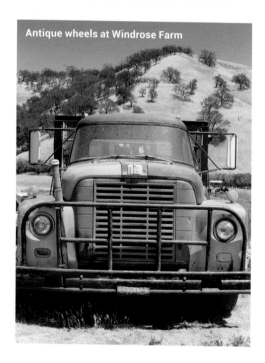

Antique wheels at Windrose Farm

ADDITIONAL FARMS IN THE AREA

Avila Valley Barn
560 Avila Beach Drive, San Luis Obispo, CA 93405; 805-595-2816, avilavalleybarn.com

Located en route to the quaint seaside community of Avila Beach, the Avila Valley Barn is a popular stop for fresh-picked produce and more in the San Luis Obispo area. What started as a simple roadside farm stand in 1985 has since grown into a fully realized shopping destination featuring a bakery, deli, summer barbecue, ice-cream parlor, and sweet shop, as well as family attractions such as hayrides, a petting zoo, and seasonal U-pick—apples in later summer and pumpkins in the fall.

BeeGreen Farm
Three Rivers, CA; 559-804-6448, beegreenfarm.com; call for directions.

Situated in the town of Three Rivers right near the entrance to Sequoia National Park, BeeGreen Farm grows heirloom fruits and boasts a stunning location about halfway between Los Angeles and the Bay Area. The farmhouse sleeps up to eight people, and guests are invited to experience farm life or simply use the home as a jumping-off point to explore the Sierra Nevada mountain range.

Bravo Farms
36005 I-99, Traver, CA 93673; 559-897-4634, bravofarms.com

Bravo Farms' Traver location (there are three others in the Central Valley) beckons I-99 travelers with multiple signs promoting cheese and wine tasting, candy, ice cream, and more. And while it would be easy to dismiss as just another tourist trap, this roadside attraction exceeds expectations with nifty novelties such as a creaky seven-story treehouse and an elevated minigolf course, as well as excellent barbecue and locally brewed beer. With plenty of outdoor seating and interesting nooks and crannies to explore, this is a worthwhile stop for both antsy kids and hungry (and thirsty) adults.

Carmel Lavender Farm

Carmel Valley, CA; 800-949-2645, carmellavender.com; call for directions.

Beekeeper and lavender grower John Russo offers workshops on the topics of beekeeping, distillation, and soap making at his Carmel Valley farm. He also rents out an off-the-grid, 400-square-foot "tiny house" on the property for those in search of a peaceful, secluded retreat. The house sleeps four in a queen bed and a sleeping loft, is completely solar-powered, and has its own well.

Country Flat Farm

Big Sur, CA; 831-624-2894, countryflatfarm.com; call for directions.

The Eichorn family has been farming in an area of the Big Sur mountains known as Palo Colorado since 1984, growing a variety of fruits and vegetables year-round and even supporting a small community CSA. The family now focuses on growing Meyer lemons (which are sold at the Earthbound Farm Stand; see page 70) and producing honey. The Eichorns offer beekeeping workshops and organic gardening classes and rent out one-bedroom standalone cottages on their gorgeous property.

Crystal Bay Farm

40 Zils Road, Watsonville, CA 95076; 831-724-4137, crystalbayfarm.com

Wife and husband Lori and Jeff open their organic Watsonville farm to visitors for educational farm stays and communal women's retreats June–October. Sleeping accommodations are under an open canopy outdoors, or guests are welcome to bring their own tents. They also offer seasonal U-pick berries and flowers.

Dare 2 Dream Farms

Near Lompoc, CA; 805-735-3233, dare2dreamfarms.com. Visit the website for directions.

This family-owned farm just outside of Lompoc helps budding urban and suburban farmers set up their own backyard chicken coops. They sell various breeds of chickens and custom-made coops, and even deliver throughout Central and Southern California. Dare 2 Dream also serves as an educational resource by offering courses to those interested in chicken keeping, and welcomes visitors to the farm by appointment.

Esalen

55000 CA 1, Big Sur, CA 93920; 831-667-3000, esalen.org

With its supreme location on the Big Sur Coast and well-established reputation as a divine retreat for the mind and body, Esalen is a place that everyone should visit at some point. What many people don't realize is that, in addition to offering yoga and meditation workshops, hot mineral springs, massage therapy, and personal retreats, Esalen also maintains a farm and garden. Visitors can participate in farming workshops, volunteer days, and apprenticeships.

The FarmStead

2323 Old Coast Highway Road, Gaviota, CA 93117; 805-689-1450, farmsteadca.com

This organic farm located just off Highway 101 between Gaviota and Buellton sells its produce daily out of its vintage barn and offers pick-your-own strawberries, raspberries, snap peas, and pumpkins in season. The FarmStead is also home to free-roaming pigs, donkeys, llamas, and goats, who enjoy being fed leftover vegetable scraps by visitors.

Jack Creek Farms

5000 CA 46 W., Templeton, CA 93465; 805-239-1915, jackcreekfarms.com

A popular destination for families between Paso Robles and Templeton, Jack Creek Farms features a country store where you can buy farm-fresh goodies such as apple cider slushies, pomegranate juice granitas, honey, and fudge. The farm also offers a slew of activities and attractions to keep kids entertained, including a toddler hay maze, farm animals, water pump barrels, a wooden train play structure, and a pumpkin patch in the fall. Jack Creek also offers U-pick gardens for most of their crops, including berries, stone fruit, tomatoes, and flowers. Call ahead or check the website to find out what's in season.

Jackson Family Farm Stay

40200 Road 28, Kingsburg, CA 93631; 559-387-4122, organic-farmstay.com

Much like at nearby Naylor's Organic (see page 85), the Jackson family operates an organic farm and opens their home to farm-stay guests. They've even been known to invite the Naylors' guests to the farm for the opportunity to visit their farm animals. Visitors enjoy comfortable accommodations and Continental breakfast and are invited to tour the farm, swim in the pool, soak in the hot tub, and kayak the adjacent Kings River.

Live Earth Farm

172 Litchfield Lane, Watsonville, CA 95076; 831-763-2448, liveearthfarm.net

This 75-acre organic farm in the Green Valley grows a diverse selection of fruits and vegetables year-round. Eager to educate the community about sustainable farming, Live Earth is open to visitors on a regular basis, offering children's programs, farm tours, school field trips, home-school days, and special events, and has a CSA program.

The Luffa Farm

1457 Willow Road, Nipomo, CA 93444; 805-343-0883, theluffafarm.com

This farm and gift shop a few miles off US 101 answers the question that many have asked: "What exactly is a luffa sponge, and where does it come from?" Yes, the farm grows heirloom luffas, a type of gourd that is dried and peeled to produce the popular skin-sloughing bath tool. Free tours are offered, but call ahead or check the website to ensure the farm is open at the time of your visit.

Margarita Adventures

22719 El Camino Real, Santa Margarita, CA 93453; 805-438-3120, margarita-adventures.com

At first glance, Margarita Adventures may seem like just another outfit targeted toward outdoorsy thrill-seekers with its zip-lining and kayaking packages. But the company boasts a very special location on the historic Santa Margarita Ranch, which has an intriguing geological and agricultural history and is currently home to an expansive sustainable cattle-ranching operation. Margarita's standard zip line tour lasts about 2 hours; this includes a half-hour ride to and from the course through the 14,000-acre property, during which the driver informs riders about how the region's unique geography enriches the ranch's soil and how that allows sister operation Ancient Peaks Winery to grow a diverse array of wine grapes. After the tour, guests can sample the results at the tasting room just across the street.

McKellar Family Farms

32988 Road 164, Ivanhoe, CA 93235; 559-798-0557,
mckellarfamilyfarms.com

A family-owned citrus farm since 1927, McKellar Family Farms offers
behind-the-scenes farm tours for large groups and rents out the
historic buildings on the property as special-event venues. Individuals
and smaller groups are welcome to visit the farm and try out the
orange grove maze (said to be the only one in the United States) on
weekdays, but should call ahead to make a reservation.

Pasolivo

8530 Vineyard Drive, Paso Robles, CA 93446; 805-227-0186, pasolivo.com

Much like nearby Kiler Ridge (see page 82), Pasolivo opens its ranch
to the public for tours and to taste its extra-virgin olive oil. The orchards
are planted on 45 acres of beautiful rolling hills, and visitors can
explore the ranch, check out the on-site olive press, sample oils and
specialty foods, and try out Pasolivo's bath and beauty products.

R&G Land and Cattle Co.

22100 Airline Highway, Paicines, CA 95043; 831-389-4263, ranchstay.net

Started as a personal family retreat near Pinnacles National Park,
R&G has since grown into a diverse agricultural operation encompassing a cattle ranch, a horse training facility, and an award-winning
organic olive oil production facility. Several lodging options are also
offered on the ranch, including private cottages and a bunkhouse
that sleeps 15.

Rosa Brothers Dairy

10090 Second Ave., Hanford, CA 93230; 559-582-8825, rosabrothers.com

This family-owned and -operated dairy is devoted to producing the
freshest, best-tasting milk possible from its herd of cows. One-hour
tours are offered by reservation and cover proper animal care, sustainable water management, the milking process, and more. Visitors
also get the opportunity to pet a baby calf and practice on a milking
simulator. Afterward, you'll want to take home a glass bottle of the
dairy's incredibly creamy, delicious milk.

Sweet Pea Farm

Arroyo Grande, CA; tinyurl.com/sweetpeafarm

This small organic family farm enjoys the near-perfect microclimate of the Central Coast and is conveniently located near Pismo Beach and Oceano Dunes State Recreation Area. Sweet Pea grows veggies, herbs, and raspberries and is also home to chickens, pigs, and canines. Visitors are welcome to either bring their own tents to camp on the property or stay in the farm's guest cabin (at the time of publication, a "glamping" dome was in the works, as well), and all guests get to enjoy fresh eggs from the hens, produce from the gardens and warm hospitality from owners Suzy and Lorraine.

V6 Ranch

70410 Parkfield Coalinga Road, Parkfield, CA 93451; 805-463-2493, v6ranch.com

This dude ranch in the Central Valley offers horseback riding, cattle drives, and a "cowboy academy," which includes lessons in cattle wrangling, trail riding, and barrel racing. But just because V6 celebrates the rugged life on the ranch doesn't mean guests have to rough it; the comfortable lodge offers all the comforts of home and then some, including wine tasting, massage, and a pool and spa. Various events and packages for all ages are offered at the ranch; visit the website for a full calendar of upcoming events.

Work Family Ranch

75893 Ranchita Canyon Road, San Miguel, CA 93451; 805-467-3362, workranch.com

The Work family (yes, that's their name) have been opening their 12,000-acre ranch to visitors for many years, making them pioneers of the agritourism movement in California. Guests can visit for a day of horseback riding, to attend youth horse camps, or to enjoy a farm stay in the guesthouse when it is available.

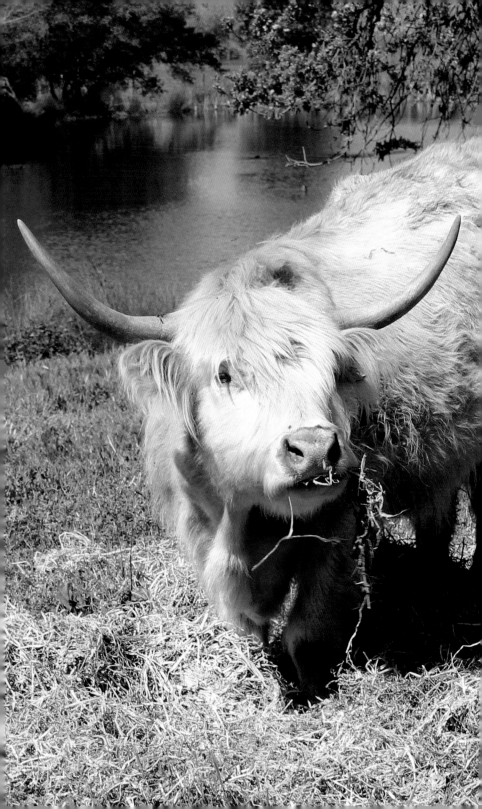

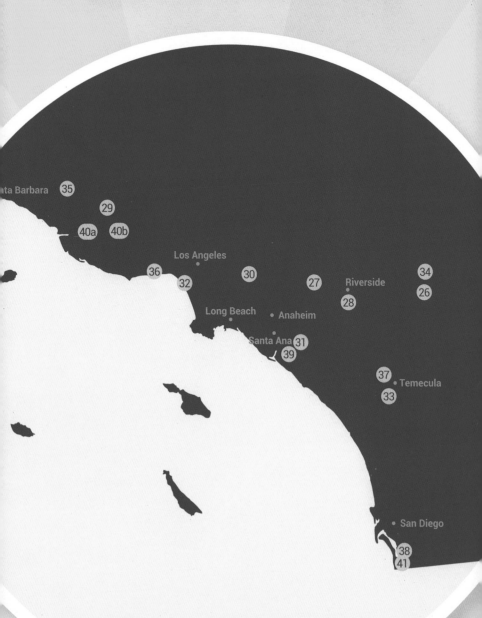

Southern
CALIFORNIA

Santa Barbara 35

29

40a 40b

Los Angeles

36

32

30

Los Angeles

27

Riverside 34

26

28

Long Beach

Anaheim

Santa Ana 31

39

37 • Temecula

33

• San Diego

38
41

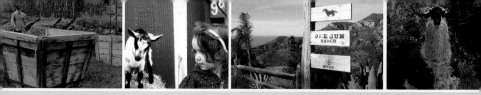

FARMS TO VISIT IN SOUTHERN CALIFORNIA

123 FARM AT HIGHLAND SPRINGS RESORT

10600 Highland Springs Ave., Beaumont, CA 92223; 951-845-1151, 123farm.com. Open year-round, but call ahead to confirm.

WHAT THEY OFFER Camps, dining, gift shop, seasonal events, tours

CHERRY VALLEY IS A TRADITIONALLY RURAL, but steadily developing, community in the foothills of the San Bernardino Mountains. The town's landmark Highland Springs Resort has a rich history dating back to the 1800s; it was known as Smith Station and operated as a stagecoach stop before being developed into a health resort in 1927. That commitment to holistic living continues today, as the rustic resort now operates the organic 123 Farm and is dedicated to preserving the natural landscape of the area for native wildlife. The name was inspired by Southern California's mild climate, which essentially consists of three seasons—spring, summer, and an extra-long fall—and lends itself to growing crops year-round. The resort and farm are just about 15 minutes down the hill from Oak Glen, so it makes sense to stop by if you're in the area picking apples in the fall. And 123 Farm is a destination in its own right every spring when it hosts the popular Lavender Festival,

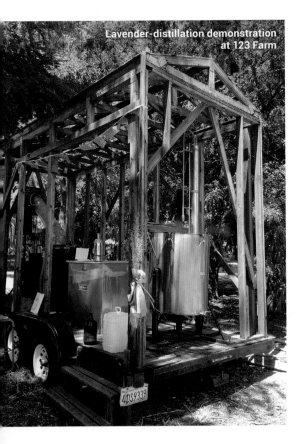

Lavender-distillation demonstration at 123 Farm

typically held over two weekends in June, as well as during other seasonal events in the spring and fall.

A huge draw for Southern Californians seeking responsibly made and grown local goods, beautiful natural surroundings, and, of course, the soothing aromatherapeutic benefits of the lavender plant, the Lavender Festival attracts large crowds. But good organization and an abundance of open space make it much more manageable than other seasonal festivals of its ilk. Another huge benefit is the generous amount of shade, as the Inland Empire in mid-June can be a pretty sweltering place. Fortunately, thick stands of mature cedar and olive trees shelter much of the festival grounds, including the large picnicking area, where attendees can sit back and listen to live music and munch on lavender-infused ice cream and pastries, or on more typical festival fare such as veggie wraps and burgers, hot dogs, sausages, and beef brisket sandwiches. There are plenty of shopping opportunities, as well, including an "organic gallery" of shops selling teas, honey, olive oil, and skin care products made on the farm.

Complimentary activities included with festival admission include seminars on topics such as naturopathy, beekeeping, edible flowers, and cooking with lavender, as well as several lavender distillation demonstrations a day, which include a brief lecture and Q&A session about how to successfully grow lavender in SoCal's varying climates. For an additional fee, visitors can take a horse-drawn wagon tour through the blooming lavender fields. The appeal of this prospect will vary depending on how hot and sunny it is, as the fields, while lovely, don't offer any shade. The farm hosts other seasonal activities throughout the year, as well, including a sheep-shearing event and weekly "grill nights" in the spring, a late-summer sausage-and-beer festival, and an olive-and-wine fair in the fall.

In addition to growing countless varieties of lavender, 123 Farm maintains a couple of acres of dozens of organic vegetable crops as an ongoing experiment in what grows best in this environment. It is also home to sheep and chickens, whose meat and eggs, along with the farm's produce, supply Highland Springs Resort's Grand Oak Steakhouse & Bar, and there are plans to start raising pastured cattle, as well. Sustainable farming methods are incorporated throughout 123's growing and animal husbandry practices: cover cropping, compost tea, and animal manure enrich the soil, and additional water-saving and regenerative practices such as mulching and no-till farming are being put into place, as well. The farm tests its soil regularly, produces all of its own fertilizer and compost, and irrigates from a natural on-site reservoir, ensuring that everything that goes into growing its crops is unadulterated by chemicals of any kind.

Every summer, 123 Farm hosts both day camp and overnight programs for kids from preschool through 12th grade. Camp instructors are the same employees who run the farm year-round, and they offer a comprehensive education in organic and sustainable farming. While drop-in visitors are generally welcome to come visit the farm, the grounds are closed to the public when camps or special events are taking place, so visitors should call ahead to confirm. Private tours can also be scheduled for a modest fee by calling or e-mailing the farm.

27 **AMY'S FARM**

7698 Eucalyptus Ave., Ontario, CA 91762; 844-426–9732, amysfarm.com; open year-round; closed Sundays

WHAT THEY OFFER Classes and workshops, farm stand, tours, volunteer opportunities

WHEN YOU CONSIDER THE AMOUNT of open, rural space surrounding Amy's Farm, it's both surprising and disheartening to consider that the small farm serves a community that is considered a food desert. Located in southern Ontario near the border of Chino, a city known as much for cow dairies as for a state prison facility, Amy's Farm sits on a piece of land that is zoned for condominiums in a rapidly developing area of the Inland Empire. The 10-acre property is leased and operated by a 501(c)(3) nonprofit organization with the goal of eventually purchasing the land so it can be protected as an agricultural preserve. In the meantime, Farmer Randy and his team serve as dedicated stewards of the land while cultivating an incredible connection with families in Riverside and San Bernardino County by hosting school field trips, private group tours, "science of farming" classes for school-age kids, and "parent and me" programs for very young children. The farm also welcomes casual visitors Monday–Saturday and operates a self-serve farm stand that operates on the honor system.

While Amy's Farm is not an overtly religious organization, the mission of its leaders is clearly informed by Christian values such as self-discipline, neighborliness, and service. The farm is dedicated to the practice of polyculture, which means growing diverse groupings of crops together in the same areas, rotating crops after each harvest, attracting beneficial insects, and generally fostering a naturally diverse ecosystem where plants can thrive, thereby eliminating the need for unnatural interventions such as pesticides and genetic modification of seed. Farmer Randy, with many decades of farming experience under his belt, is quick to point out that this is nothing more than a back-to-basics approach to growing food that emulates what Mother Nature has already mastered.

Like any proper diversified agricultural operation, Amy's Farm doesn't just grow crops but raises animals, too. Tours of the farm for both schoolchildren and small groups last an hour to an hour and a half and include feeding the pigs, chickens, geese, and ducks, as well as milking a cow and visiting the goats and horses. The animals are humanely raised and fed an organic, non-GMO diet of feed and veggies from the farm, and their eggs and meat can be purchased at the produce stand.

In addition to land preservation and community development, Amy's Farm is devoted to education. The highly interactive farm tours are designed to empower children and adults to grow their own food sustainably. Kids are encouraged to start edible gardens, at home or at their schools, churches, or other institutions. What's more, the farm's educational programs place as much emphasis on emotional health as they do on physical well-being. To that end, Amy's Farm employs an on-site licensed marriage and family therapist and regularly opens the facility to disabled groups and veterans.

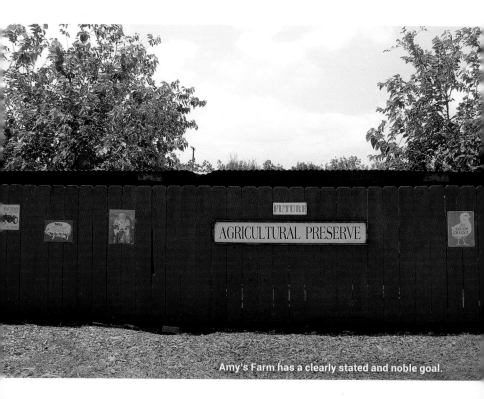

Amy's Farm has a clearly stated and noble goal.

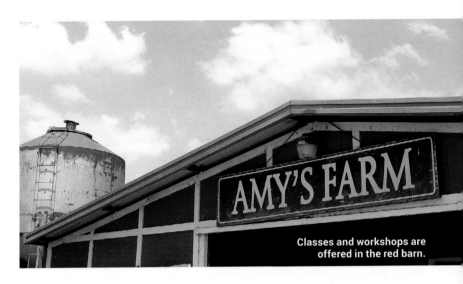

Classes and workshops are offered in the red barn.

If you'd like to tour Amy's Farm, plan to book several weeks in advance so you can choose a date when the farm isn't overrun with school groups. Workshops geared toward everyone from toddlers to high school kids are offered year-round; find a list and description of upcoming topics, which could be anything from simple farm machines to dissecting a sheep's heart, on the website. And if you want to simply drop in for a casual visit, be advised that spring and fall are the busiest times of year, and the afternoon is usually a quieter time of day to visit. The farm also welcomes volunteers of all ages. Volunteers are asked to attend an orientation meeting with Farmer Randy, and can then enjoy flexible hours and an ongoing, hands-on course in sustainable farming and self-sufficiency.

28 CALIFORNIA CITRUS STATE HISTORIC PARK

9400 Dufferin Ave., Riverside, CA 92504; 951-780-6222, tinyurl.com/californiacitrusshp; open year-round

WHAT THEY OFFER Gift shop, hiking, museum, tasting, tours

THERE'S NO OTHER PLACE IN CALIFORNIA quite like the Citrus State Historic Park, which is unique in the sense that it's the only state park that grows edibles and, better yet, encourages visitors to eat them. The park is in the historic Arlington Heights neighborhood in a scenic rural section of the city of Riverside. While the park is open year-round, the best time to visit is in the winter, when temperatures are cool to mild, the air is clean, and pretty much all the fruit is ripe for the picking. Depending on what direction you approach the park from, you may be greeted on your way by a cheery replica of an old-fashioned roadside fruit stand adorned with a giant orange, located at the corner of Van Buren Boulevard and Dufferin Avenue.

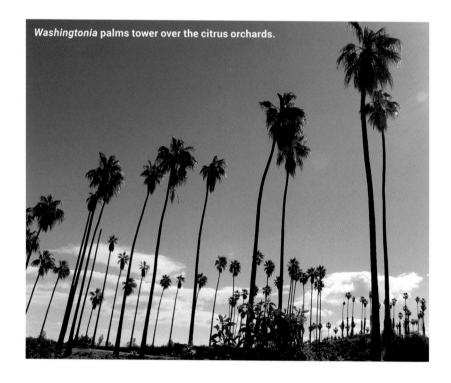

Washingtonia **palms tower over the citrus orchards.**

California Citrus State Park covers 377 acres, 200 of which are overseen by the commercial citrus-farming operation Gless Ranch, which picks the fruit, maintains the groves, and gives 60% of its revenue back to the state park. The remaining acreage is devoted to growing more than 75 different varietals of citrus and preserving a piece of Southern California's rapidly vanishing citrus industry. Because this is a nonprofit, all the fruit grown in this area is offered to visitors who take the tour, school groups, senior centers, and food banks.

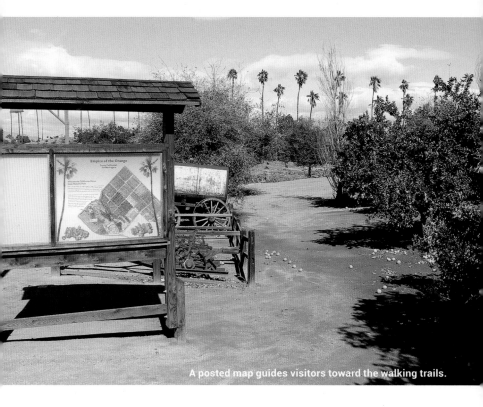

A posted map guides visitors toward the walking trails.

The park is open to the public seven days a week, and visitors are encouraged to grab a self-guided tour map and explore the park's accessible trails through terraced citrus groves, avocado orchards, eucalyptus forests, and towering *Washingtonia* palms. But you're better off coming on the weekend for a free docent-guided tour (call ahead to let them know you're coming), which includes all-you-can-eat orange, tangerine, mandarin, kumquat, pomelo, and grapefruit tasting that's sure to leave you puckered up and not at all deficient in vitamin C. The icing on the cake? You get to collect fruit to take home over the course of the tour—you'll leave with a bulging bag full of obscure and delicious types of fruit you'd never find at the supermarket, along with reliable favorites such as blood oranges, navels, and Satsuma mandarins. Of course, you're not just in this for the free food; you're here to learn about citrus farming. And in that regard, you won't be disappointed, as the park's docents will teach you all about the history of the citrus industry and the land, how the trees are cultivated and maintained, and the differences between the dozens of varietals of fruit grown here.

The tour may last anywhere from 45 minutes to an hour and a half, depending on which guide you get and how engaged your group is, and covers about a mile of trails, with a bit of elevation change and some tracking through dense groves to make you feel a little bit rugged. Afterward, you'll want to visit the on-site museum and gift shop. The small but impressive museum gives a comprehensive look at the history of citrus farming, from traveling the Silk Road in 500 BC to ancient Rome to its arrival in the Americas in the 1500s to the rise of Californian agriculture in the 1800s. Interactive elements make the exhibits engaging for children as well as adults, but the truth is, young ones will probably be most drawn to the gift shop, which offers a nicely curated selection of citrus-scented soaps, tchotchkes, toys, and sweet treats, along with an incredible array of classic packing-crate labels.

TIPS Be prepared to get sticky. Your tour guide will provide plastic gloves for tasting the citrus slices and segments provided over the course of the tour, but they're juicy and sticky, so you might want to bring your own napkins or wet wipes. Also, be aware that picking any fruit without permission is strictly prohibited, so ask your docent to pick anything you're interested in tasting, or wait for his or her go-ahead to pick.

29 CHIVAS SKIN CARE AND GOAT FARM

2220 Bardsdale Ave., Fillmore, CA 93015; 805-727-3121, chivasskincare.com/farm-events. Open by appointment for tours and several times a year for seasonal events.

WHAT THEY OFFER Classes and workshops, gift shop, seasonal events, tours

CHIVAS SKIN CARE IS A LABOR OF LOVE run entirely from a small family farm in the rural town of Fillmore in inland Ventura County. *Chivas* means "female goats" in Spanish, and mother-daughter team Donna Johanson and Lauren Johanson Jones handcraft gentle soaps made from the milk of their herd of French Alpine goats. The skin care line also includes bath salts, body butters, eye cream, lip balm, and other nourishing treats for the skin. The products are scented with intoxicating essential oil blends such as lavender-mint, patchouli-cedar, lemon-eucalyptus, and rose-geranium, and with herbs sourced from the Johansons' own garden.

Because this is a private home, the Chivas farm isn't generally open to the public. But several times a year, Donna and Lauren open their modest, 1-acre homestead to the public for seasonally themed events, offering educational tours of the farm and soap-making facilities; homemade cookies and beverages; outdoor "farm games"; and photo ops with goats, pigs, tortoises, and calves. You can also schedule a class field trip or private group tour of the farm; tours generally last about an hour and can be customized to suit the visitors' interests and age range.

Chivas's "open farm" events have pretty broad appeal. If you're a conscientious consumer, particularly of beauty products, you'll come away with a better understanding of how those products are made and, in particular, what sets strictly nature-derived ingredients apart from those manufactured in a lab. Inside the soap-making facility, the scent of essentials oils alone will send you into a state of deep relaxation as Donna and Lauren walk you through the entire process, from milking to molding, and give you an appreciation for just how much labor goes into making soap by hand without adding any water, mineral oil, or artificial fragrances and preservatives. If you're an aspiring urban or suburban homesteader, you'll observe firsthand the reality of keeping farm animals and growing crops on a small (at least by farm standards) lot. And if you're a kid—or a kid at heart—you'll simply have a blast searching for eggs in the chicken coop, feeding pigs and tortoises, and maybe even learning how to milk a goat. Spring is probably the best time to visit because that's when the baby goats are born, and they're awfully cute and cuddly, even when they're practically chewing your clothes off.

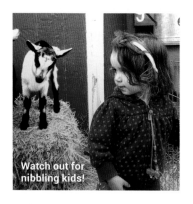

Watch out for nibbling kids!

Because the farm's primary business is marketing and selling the Chivas Skin Care line, all events feature an on-site cottage, where you can purchase any of their products. Holiday-themed events, such as the Mother's Day tea party, Father's Day garden party, and fall festival, are held throughout the year. And every December, the farm hosts a festive holiday boutique, during which they expand their offerings to include design-inspired farm tools, handmade jewelry, and other gift-y items. All events offer guests the option of taking farm and soap-making tours, as well as occasional hands-on activities such as DIY sugar scrub, bath salt, and massage oil workshops.

To stay apprised of upcoming events at the Chivas goat farm, follow Chivas Skin Care on Facebook (facebook.com/chivasskincare) or visit the website. And if you're interested in trying out the products in the meantime, Chivas Skin Care items are sold in certain stores and various SoCal farmers markets, as well as online. Check the website for more information.

TIPS When you visit the farm, stock up on your favorite soap fragrance blends at the on-site shop, where unwrapped soaps are sold at a discount. And if you're visiting with kids, ask if they can visit the chicken coop to collect eggs.

30 EARTHWORKS FARM

1210 Lerma Road, South El Monte, CA 91733; 626-374-3504,
earthworksfarmgarden.org. Open year-round; check website for days and hours.
Park in the lot for Special Events Area B.

WHAT THEY OFFER CSA, farm stand, tours, volunteer opportunities

LOCATED IN THE IMPOVERISHED COMMUNITY of South El Monte,
about 15 minutes east of downtown Los Angeles and in the shadow
of the Pomona Freeway, Earthworks is the quintessential urban farm.
Nearly 5 acres of organic fields and orchards feed hundreds of families
every week, and the farm's location on a natural watershed allows for the
cultivation of a diverse array of fruits and vegetables, including tropical
fruits, grapes, several types of citrus, avocados, and many vegetables
that are popular in Asian and Central and South American cuisines. The
land is part of the Whittier Narrows Recreation Area, a 14,000-acre park
that flanks the freeway and features lakes for boating and fishing, a golf
course, an equestrian center, picnic areas, sports fields, and a bunch of
other opportunities for outdoor fun. Unfortunately, despite this wealth of
outdoor-recreation opportunities and incredible resource for locally grown
produce, the local population is considered to be among the unhealthiest
in the state of California. But the Earthworks team are doing their best to
change that with the farm's community outreach endeavors, including
harvest tours, a produce stand, a CSA program, and open volunteer hours.

Volunteering at Earthworks is a simple and rewarding process. All ages
and skill levels are welcome, and the schedule is flexible. Simply e-mail
or call ahead and you'll be invited down to the farm to lend a hand. Your
duties may include weeding, planting, or hauling wheelbarrows of garden
waste to the compost piles. Be sure to wear a hat and sunscreen, long
pants, and closed-toe shoes, and expect it to be hot in the summer. Kids,
naturally, must be supervised by an adult to make sure they don't end
up trampling seedlings or accidentally pulling up a whole crop. But they
will no doubt enjoy visiting the Loquat Spot, a shady corner of the farm
with hay bales to sit on and a bench swing hanging from a canopy of tree
branches. Volunteers not only get to take home fresh veggies, but those

who donate a minimum number of work hours every week also get their own garden bed at the farm and seeds to plant, maintain, and harvest. When you consider the price of real estate in Los Angeles and the fact that most of the area's community gardens have multiyear waiting lists, this is quite an incentive indeed.

But the main reward of working on the Earthworks Farm comes from the experience itself. If you don't have the opportunity to keep your own garden at home, you may very well find a deep satisfaction in tasks like adding garden waste to a growing pile of compost, pushing wheelbarrows full of freshly picked veggies to the produce stand, or unearthing the root ball of a particularly stubborn weed. This is what it feels like to work the land, and Earthworks happily makes the opportunity available to all who want to get their hands dirty. The fact that the dull roar of the freeway provides steady background noise adds to the novelty of the experience.

If you'd like to simply explore the farm without putting in manual labor, you can sign up for one of the regular harvest tours, which are offered to school groups, families, and individuals at a very reasonable charge. If you live in the area, sign up for the CSA; members enjoy a weekly box of whatever is in season. Earthworks also operates a produce stand on Saturdays, and casual visitors are even welcome to come to the farm during the week to purchase fresh produce—so fresh that a farmer will go into the field to fulfill your order on the spot. The prices are purposely affordable to serve the local community, and considering how conveniently the farm is to the freeway, stopping by is pretty much a no-brainer if you're driving through the area.

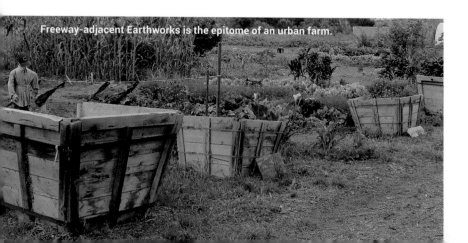
Freeway-adjacent Earthworks is the epitome of an urban farm.

31 FOOD + FARM LAB AT OC GREAT PARK

Irvine, CA; 866-829-3829, ocgp.org, alegriafresh.com; open year-round.
Visit the website for directions and a calendar of events.

WHAT THEY OFFER Classes and workshops, farmers market, kids' activities and events, tours

IT HAS TAKEN A FEW YEARS for Orange County Great Park in Irvine to find its footing, but devoting several acres of the vast regional park to innovative agricultural pursuits was definitely a wise plan. Encompassing a total area of 1,300 acres, Great Park is the former site of a Marine Corps Air Station and has added attractions and landscaping over the last several years to attract visitors from all over Orange and Los Angeles Counties. However, much of the area still feels barren and unfinished (the lack of shade can be particularly irksome on a hot summer day), and the park's development has been plagued with controversy over possible misuse of public funds. Despite all that, it's still a worthwhile place to visit, thanks in large part to the expertly designed and implemented Farm + Food Lab on the premises.

Great Park will eventually devote even more land to agriculture and community gardens, which makes sense given the amount of open space, ample sunshine, and agricultural history of the area (before it was an air base, this was a prolific lima bean field). In the meantime, the 1-acre Food + Farm Lab serves as a highly interactive and educational demonstration site for sustainable urban agriculture. The garden is staffed by University of California Cooperative Extension Master Gardeners and is open seven days a week. Free, half-hour guided tours can be arranged, but visitors are also welcome to drop by for self-guided tours. The garden showcases concepts such as vertical gardening, themed raised-bed gardens, and fruit orchards, and informational signage throughout goes into detail about topics such as composting, beneficial versus harmful insects, fertilizers, crop rotation, year-round gardening in Southern California, and even unconventional ideas such as straw-bale gardening. There are plenty of hands-on features to engage kids, as well, such as a large, open worm compost bin, magnifying glasses to look closely at plants and insects, interactive quizzes, hopscotch, and a chicken coop. In addition to tours, Food + Farm Lab's Master Gardeners host free workshops throughout the year on topics such as preserving, gardening with kids, and seasonal cooking, as well as special programs for little ones, such as story time and drum circles.

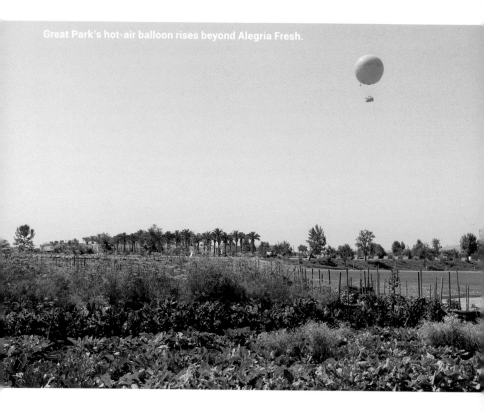

Great Park's hot-air balloon rises beyond Alegria Fresh.

But Food + Farm Lab isn't the only exciting agricultural endeavor happening in Great Park: directly across a big parking lot lies the high-yield microfarm site of Alegria Fresh. The company uses vertical hydroponic growing systems, as well as GardenSoxx, which hold the farm's carefully formulated organic soil mixture in patented mesh enclosures that are placed aboveground, much like raised beds, but are especially moisture-retaining and weed-resistant. It's a smart and innovative system, if not particularly pretty to look at. But the farm itself is still lovely, filled with lush edible flower bushes, towering sunflowers, and perennial kale plants that have grown so tall they look like palm trees. Casual visitors are welcome to walk through and explore the gardens, but if you bring kids along, you will be politely asked to hold them by the hand while on the premises. If you want to learn more about the farm's extreme efficiency of production and mission to train urban farmers about sustainable agriculture, expert-led tours of the farm can be booked for a suggested donation. Alegria Fresh also sells its innovative planters and vertical gardening systems to home gardeners and small-scale farmers.

Last but not least, Great Park maintains its own organic farm. The produce is sold at the on-site Sunday Farmers Market and donated to local food banks. Additional attractions at the park include a merry-go-round, a playground, and a hot-air balloon that rises 400 feet to give riders a 360-degree view of Orange County.

> **TIP** OC Great Park doesn't have a street address but is located just east of I-5 at the Sand Canyon exit. The website provides detailed directions from wherever you're coming from. Parking in the lot for Farm + Food Lab places you fairly close to the visitor center, balloon ride, and playground. From there, it's a short walk to the Alegria Fresh farm and farmers market.

32 KISS THE GROUND GARDEN

681 N. Venice Blvd., Los Angeles, CA 90291; kisstheground.com; open year-round. Sign up for newsletter to stay informed about upcoming events.

WHAT THEY OFFER Classes and workshops, special events, volunteer opportunities

KISS THE GROUND IS RUN BY A GROUP of people that may well represent the archetype that many associate with Venice Beach. The organization was co-founded by Ryland Engelhart, owner of mystical raw-food emporium Café Gratitude, and musician Finian Makepeace and is overseen by a passionate young group of hip, healthy, and attractive creative types you'd expect to find living in this bohemian beach community. Stereotypes and preconceived notions aside, these "cool kids" are doing incredible—and important—work.

Kiss the Ground has a stated mission "to inspire global participation in the restoration of our precious soil." And if you spend any time talking to co-founder Finian, he will gladly inform you about the importance of rebuilding and restoring the humus in our cultivated land's topsoil, which acts like a sponge to retain moisture and return carbon to the soil, as opposed to releasing it into the atmosphere. It's a pretty heady topic involving microbiology, but the upshot is this: You can either grow plants in a way that releases carbon into the atmosphere or in a way that keeps carbon in the soil. Needless to say, the latter option is much better.

When they got started, Finian and his team of activists at Kiss the Ground had a passion for their extraordinarily worthy cause but no land, so they started by planting temporary demonstration gardens around the scrappy beach community to build awareness and support for their cause. And it paid off: thanks to its founders' dedicated policy efforts, Kiss the Ground has managed to create something more permanent on city land. Their regenerative garden is located at the Venice Arts Plaza, a historic site that encompasses Venice's former city hall, police station, and jail, and is now home to nonprofit arts organizations Beyond Baroque and the Social and Public Art Resource Center (SPARC). Kiss the Ground's demonstration garden is currently a work in progress, with fruit trees, raised vegetable garden beds, a greenhouse, a children's garden, and a cob pizza oven already in place, and a gray-water irrigation system, shade trees, and more edible gardens still in store.

NEARBY ATTRACTION Chocovivo

(Full disclosure: A good portion of this book was written while the author indulged in salted brown butter chocolate chip cookies and thick, rich sipping chocolate at the café's hand-carved communal wooden table.)

Chocovivo is Los Angeles' only bean-to-bar chocolate maker, serving direct-trade, rustic, stone-ground chocolate that will have you hooked after just one nibble. The café has the feel of a neighborhood gathering spot; much of its clientele are repeat visitors who settle in and make themselves at home with a plate of tamales or a deeply satisfying mug of dark hot chocolate. But first-timers feel welcome, as well, and owner Patricia Tsai and her employees are happy to explain the origins and health benefits of cacao, as well as the chocolate-making process, which occurs right in the shop's kitchen. Patricia sources all of her cacao beans directly from a farm in Tabasco, Mexico, which she visits regularly to understand the growing process and cultivate a relationship with the farmers. In addition to dark chocolate drinks and bars flavored with various nuts, fruits, and spices, Chocovivo serves tamales made by a neighborhood chef several days a week, as well as homemade ice cream, pastries, and coffee. The café is open late (presenting a convenient dessert option for the many restaurants within walking distance) and offers free Wi-Fi.

12469 W. Washington Blvd., Culver City, CA 90066; 310-845-6259, chocovivo.com; open daily

The urban farm's maintenance and development is overseen by UC Master Gardener and permaculture expert Lauren Tucker, who can often be found tending to the crops. Garden workdays are open to the community and, in keeping with the neighborhood vibe, often begin with a morning yoga class. In addition to volunteer opportunities, Kiss the Ground holds regular educational events covering compost making, permaculture design, fruit tree pruning, and other topics. Some workshops charge a fee, while others offer free training for volunteers. Other events, both for free and for fundraising, such as garden concerts and farm-to-table dinners, are also held throughout the year. Anyone interested can stay up-to-date on all of Kiss the Ground's goings-on by signing up for their newsletter. And because this is public land, casual visitors are always welcome to drop by for a self-guided tour—the gardens offer a welcoming and unexpected oasis on busy Venice Boulevard.

33 MORNING SONG FARM

Rainbow, CA; 888-816-3335, morningsongfarm.com. Call or e-mail csa@morningsongfarm.com for directions. Farm stays are offered year-round.

WHAT THEY OFFER Classes and workshops, CSA, lodging, tours

MORNING SONG FARM'S DONNA BUONO invites you to join her menagerie for a peaceful, bountiful, and thoroughly comfortable stay. This hilly, 20-acre respite overlooking the Rainbow Valley is home to Donna and her family, along with a llama, goats, and cats—all full of personality—and produces an impressive amount of macadamia nuts and a diverse selection of fruits and vegetables, including rare finds such as Persian mulberries, jujubes, passion fruit, and dragon fruit, as well as eggs and honey. The whole farm is organic and overseen by Donna, partner Lance, and a handful of hardworking college kids (including Donna's son).

The Morning Song Farm Stay enterprise began with Donna simply making her guest unit available to friends and friends of friends who were craving an escape. Now the experience is available to a broader clientele through Airbnb, but Donna's spirit of generosity is still evident in the reasonable nightly rate, the well-stocked kitchen, and the immediate spirit of welcome afforded to her guests. Getting there is a bit of an adventure—the farm's entry gate is located on the exquisitely windy Rainbow Glen Road, and once you're inside, be prepared to navigate a narrow, climbing (but thankfully, paved) road to reach your front door. Fortunately, Donna provides detailed directions, and once you arrive, the waiting bottle of wine, outdoor hot tub, and gorgeous view of the valley will immediately compel you to kick back and make yourself at home.

Given how well Donna provides for her guests, you may not find any reason to leave the farm once you've settled in to one of the two available guest units. The one-bedroom unit is smallish—best suited for one or two people—but includes everything one could need, including a fully equipped kitchen with fresh veggies, honey, and eggs from the farm; coffee and cream; butter; olive oil; and other pantry staples, as well as snacks like yogurt, chips, and salsa. The unit also includes satellite TV and a collection of DVDs. If you do decide to venture out, Donna and Lance can make recommendations for nearby places to eat and activities such as strawberry picking at Kenny's or wine tasting at Roadrunner Winery, both located just down the road. A two-bedroom unit that sleeps up to four adults was recently added to the farm, and includes all of the amenities of the first, along with its own fenced-in chicken garden.

In addition to operating a farm stay, Donna opens Morning Song Farm for occasional group tours that include fruit and nut tasting and a barbecue lunch. She also offers a CSA subscription to residents of many communities in coastal San Diego County. The service includes door-to-door delivery of an incredibly diverse array of Morning Song's organic produce, including standard-issue salad greens, vegetables, citrus, and avocados, along with rare and exotic fruits and nuts. What's available varies, of course, by season, and subscribers can visit the website to get an idea of what's available when, although harvest times can shift according to the vagaries of Southern California's climate. Donna even teaches cheese-making classes, which include a wood-fired pizza lunch. Contact Donna directly through the Morning Song Farm website to receive information about classes and upcoming tours.

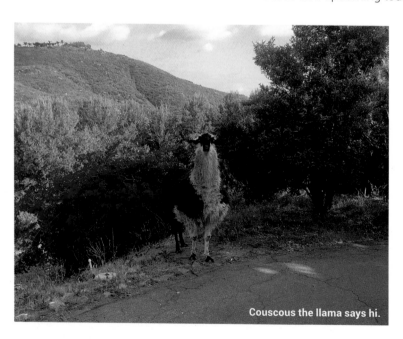

Couscous the llama says hi.

If you enjoy craft beer, you've probably heard of Stone Brewing Company. The Escondido-based brewery is hugely popular in Southern California and is particularly known for its brews with strong flavor profiles and audacious names like Arrogant Bastard, Sublimely Self Righteous, and Ruination, as well as limited releases flavored with unconventional ingredients such as hibiscus, grapefruit, and chocolate. Tours of the Escondido brewery are popular and offered daily, and the Stone Brewing World Bistro and Gardens has two San Diego County locations: one in Escondido and another in Liberty Station. But if you're looking for a low-key, ag-themed destination, head straight for Stone Farms, which is about 20 minutes south of Morning Song Farm, just off of I-15.

The farm is located down a poorly marked road and doesn't feature any obvious signage to indicate its affiliation with a major brewing company, and that's a big part of its appeal. The 19-acre property is planted with a diverse array of organically grown crops (including hops) and is home to peacocks, chickens, and quail. Order a pint (or fill a growler) at the on-site bar and store, and then simply wander the grounds, enjoying the fresh air and lovely setting of the North County Hills. If you get hungry, order a pie from the outdoor pizza oven and have a seat at one of the picnic tables. You can even hear live music from local bands if you're there on a Wednesday or Friday evening.

9928 Protea Gardens Road, Escondido, CA 92026;
stonebrewing.com/visit/stone-farms

TIP The aforementioned winding road leading to Morning Song and the narrow drive leading up to the guesthouse can be a little tricky to navigate on your first time, so plan to arrive before dark to get your bearings.

34 OAK GLEN PRESERVE AND LOS RIOS RANCHO

39611 S. Oak Glen Road, Oak Glen, CA 92399; 909-790-3698 (preserve) or 909-797-1005 (Los Rios), losriosrancho.com or wildlandsconservancy.org; open year-round

WHAT THEY OFFER Dining, gift shop, hiking, picnicking, seasonal events and activities, U-pick

OAK GLEN MAY BE BEST KNOWN as an autumn destination, when Southern Californians flock to its farm stands and apple orchards in droves for fresh-pressed cider, hayrides, U-pick apples, and addictive apple cider mini-doughnuts. But it's a gorgeous place to visit anytime of year—and thankfully, the farming community's location up in the foothills means it's usually quite a bit cooler than the flatlands, offering a welcome escape from the Inland Empire's relentless hot weather that often lasts well into fall.

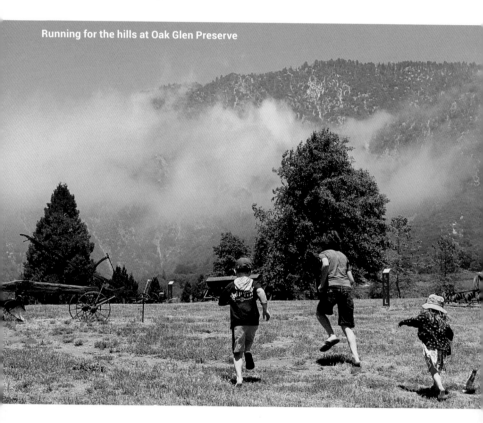

Running for the hills at Oak Glen Preserve

The Southern California Montane Botanic Garden and Children's Outdoor Discovery Center, which opened in 2014, provides a perfect excuse to visit the area anytime of year, even after the apple trees have been picked clean. Located in the midst of the scenic 2,100-acre Oak Glen Preserve, the garden's several miles of hiking trails explore ponds, streams, oak and pine forests, wetlands, grasslands, and chaparral—changes in elevation provide a heart-pumping workout as well as lovely views of the surrounding mountains and orchards.

Interactive children's quizzes interspersed along the paths make this a fun hike for kids, who will no doubt have a blast hopping from tree stump to tree stump, scrambling over boulders and splashing in the streams—just make sure they keep an eye out for the stinging nettle lining the wetlands boardwalk (it's labeled). Also, keep in mind that the gardens are surrounded by unspoiled wilderness, so mountain lions and rattlesnakes make occasional appearances here, as well.

TIPS At more than 5,000 feet in elevation, Oak Glen is invariably cooler than the flatlands. That said, it can still warm up quite a bit in the summer. On the flip side, after a winter rainstorm down below, you may find snow up here. If you go for a hike, stick to the trails to avoid poison oak and stinging nettle, and watch out for wildlife such as coyotes, rattlesnakes, bobcats, and mountain lions.

After your hike, reward yourself with fresh apple cider (hot or cold) and barbecued tri-tip sandwiches next door at Los Rios Rancho, which is a popular Oak Glen destination in its own right. The large gift shop and bakery sells apple pies, dried fruit, and other snacks, along with knickknacks and several varieties of freshly pressed apple cider, and the adjoining restaurant serves excellent barbecue. The adjacent picnic grounds are lovely, as well. Across the street in the north orchard, Los Rios offers U-pick apples and pumpkins in season, as well as fall activities such as hayrides, a corn maze, and apple cider pressing.

NEARBY ATTRACTION Law's Apple Shed and Cider Mill

Most of Oak Glen's ranches, farms, restaurants, bakeries, shops, and tourist attractions are located within a 5-mile loop on Oak Glen Road. If you're approaching Oak Glen from the east, or the Yucaipa side, one of the first businesses you'll come to is Law's Apple Shed and Cider Mill, which is smaller than the other apple stands in the area and dates back generations. This is the place to get the absolute freshest, which is to say unpasteurized, apple cider on the hill. You can also sometimes observe the apple press in action and try 35 different varieties of apples (in season). Law's Oak Glen coffee shop is next door and is renowned for its apple pie.

38392 Oak Glen Road, Oak Glen, CA 92399; 909-797-3130, lawsoakglen.com

NEARBY ATTRACTION Snow-Line Orchard

Less than 2 miles farther down the road is Snow-Line Orchard, which is just past Los Rios Rancho and set back down a long driveway from the road. Snow-Line's claims to fame are hot, fresh apple cider mini-doughnuts and a recently added hard cider tasting room. They also sell what seems like an endless variety of apples, although the orchard doesn't offer apple picking. U-pick raspberries, on the other hand, are available in season. You can also purchase three types of cider (apple, apple-raspberry, and apple-cherry) and picnic beneath what's said to be the state's oldest chestnut tree.

39400 Oak Glen Road, Oak Glen, CA 92399; 909-797-3415, snow-line.com

35 OJAI OLIVE OIL COMPANY

1811 Ladera Road, Ojai, CA 93023; 805-646-5964, ojaioliveoil.com; open year-round, Tuesday–Saturday. Tours are offered on Wednesday and Saturday. Check website for hours and detailed driving directions.

WHAT THEY OFFER Gift shop, tasting, tours

LOCATED UP A DIRT ROAD AT THE EAST END of the picturesque Ojai Valley, the 35-acre olive grove cultivated by the Ojai Olive Oil Company feels like a retreat from the rest of the world. The property is situated in a peaceful, secluded canyon that once belonged to a farmer by the name of James Leslie, who planted Spanish-variety olive trees between 1860 and 1880 with dreams of shipping olive oil to a ready market in New York City via the transcontinental railroad. Unfortunately for Mr. Leslie, harsh competition from the East Coast rendered his venture unsuccessful. He gave up on the olive oil trade in 1910, leaving the trees unmaintained and unirrigated for nearly a century, until Ojai Olive Oil founder Ronald Asquith purchased the land in 1998 to follow his dream of becoming a farmer after retiring from the corporate business world.

As luck would have it, the hardy olive trees had thrived in Ojai's ideal Mediterranean climate despite many decades of neglect. The company's first extra-virgin olive oil was produced in 2000 from fruit growing on the 140-year-old trees. At the same time, Mr. Asquith began planting additional varieties (French, Italian, Spanish, and Sicilian), in order to produce a wider range of extra-virgin olive oils, from the mild and fruity Provençale to the fresh and grassy Tuscan to the robust and peppery Andalucian.

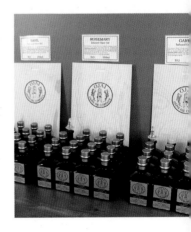

This brief history of the land and its trees comes courtesy of Ronald's wife, Alice de Dadelsen-Asquith. Since her husband died in 2013 at the age of 81, she has been sharing the duties of running the business with their son Philip Asquith in service to both her husband's legacy and to the land itself. Ojai Olive Oil became a certified organic operation in 2010, so its products are entirely free of chemical fertilizers and pesticides. To maintain a healthy ecosystem on the land for many years to come, additional permaculture principles are being implemented, as well, including digging ponds for rainwater catchment, terracing the land to minimize erosion, and composting the by-products of olive oil production to fertilize the trees. These practices are steadily improving the quality of the soil and the health of the crop, thereby keeping production strong.

Alice and Philip share the task of offering free informational talks and tasting to the public year-round on Wednesday and Saturday. The guided visits last about 30–45 minutes. Participants learn about the origin and evolution of olive oil production in California, which—despite being a relatively new industry—produces the majority of American-made olive oil. Alice or Philip also discusses organic cultivation practices, the importance of hand-picking the fruit, the yearly cycle of an olive tree, and the challenges presented by California's ongoing drought. Correct pruning procedure is another important topic; the center of a tree should be maintained in an open chalice shape that invites the sun to reach the tree's heart and encourage consistent growth. If an olive tree is well tended, it can produce for up to 1,000 years.

The visitors then move into the processing facility that houses the company's olive mill built in the Tuscan region of Italy. The state-of-the-art stainless steel machine that extracts the olive oil with a centrifuge is explained in detail. Every stage of the harvest and processing is choreographed to protect the olives from oxidation. Picking the fruit by hand allows it to be processed within 5 hours of coming off the trees, and the olives are never exposed to air to keep oxidation to a minimum. Sample the fresh-tasting results in the tasting room and gift shop located in the same WWII-era Quonset hut where the olive oils are milled, bottled, and later shipped out.

In addition to extra-virgin olive oil, the shop sells balsamic vinegars from a family-run farm in Modena, Italy. All oils and vinegars are bottled in dark blue glass to protect the contents from light and keep the product fresher longer. You can also purchase beautifully scented, olive oil–based beauty products such as lip balm, soap, and face cream, all of which make wonderful gifts if you can manage not to keep them for yourself.

36 ONE GUN RANCH

22634 Mansie Road, Malibu, CA 90265; 310-456-3810, 1gunranch.com; open to the public a few times a year

WHAT THEY OFFER School tours, seasonal events

IN MANY WAYS, ONE GUN RANCH is exactly what you would expect from a wealthy family's hobby farm in Malibu. Farm events include complimentary valet parking, the multimillion-dollar views are glorious, and the resident farmer spends a lot of time talking about the cosmic, spiritual elements of the ranch's custom-made compost. But just because the place fits a certain stereotype doesn't mean something incredible isn't happening here.

The breathtakingly beautiful property is set up in the hills and boasts stunning ocean views. It was formerly owned by Guns N' Roses drummer Matt Sorum; hence the name. But for the past several years One Gun Ranch has belonged to Ann Eysenring and Alice Bamford, who devote much of the land to biodynamic farming. Alice, in particular, boasts impressive agricultural credibility: her family has farmed organically in England for the past 40 years and her grandfather invented the backhoe. Alice and Ann have enlisted the help of experts such as head gardener Camerino Perez, who meticulously tends to the farm's seedlings and crops, and Jack McAndrews, a.k.a. "Farmer Jack," who oversees the ranch's impressive biodynamic compost-making operation. Lest you think making compost is as simple as throwing a bunch of organic matter into a pile and allowing it to decompose, Farmer Jack stands ready to explain how to take that process to a new level.

Dubbed "Super(ior) Soil," the compost is prepared on the ranch using strict biodynamic standards and principles. The recipe was developed more than 90 years ago by father of biodynamic agriculture Rudolf Steiner; it consists of two bales of alfalfa, one ton of dairy cow manure, and an infusion of homeopathic herbs and plants such as yarrow, chamomile, stinging nettle, dandelion, and valerian, which are purported to bring in energy from the cosmos and the earth to infuse the

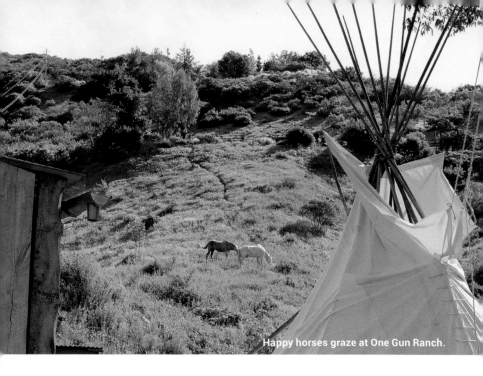

Happy horses graze at One Gun Ranch.

plants with intense healing vibrations. If that last bit sounds a little too "out there" to be believed, suffice it to say that this compost produces healthy, great-tasting crops. Jack's magic mix is used to grow all the food at One Gun Ranch and is available for sale. Sold in bulk to other farmers, it fetches $2,000 per ton, so they're obviously onto something.

You'll witness the benefits of the biodynamic compost when you visit One Gun's gardens. Although the property encompasses 22 acres, only 1 acre is used to grow crops. All plants are grown in raised beds within fenced and netted enclosures designed to keep out rabbits, deer, birds, and other garden nibblers. The small size of the farm allows the crops to be painstakingly tended, and Camerino monitors their growth closely, assiduously removing any dead or decaying plant matter to deter harmful insects and attract beneficial ones. Naturally, no pesticides or chemicals of any kind are used in biodynamic farming, so the emphasis is on keeping the plants healthy and clean and building up their natural defenses, eliminating the need for unnatural intervention. The fruits and vegetables are sold at Vintage Grocers in Malibu, as well as at a couple of other local markets and to a few restaurants.

The ranch is home to a menagerie of blissfully spoiled farm animals, including horses, goats, sheep, dogs, alpacas, pigs, and a donkey, making it a delightful place for children to visit. Even though this is a private residence, the owners are very community-minded and, to that end, make the ranch available for school tours and field trips for students ranging from preschool to college. They also host "open farm" events several times a year. Visit the website or contact the ranch directly to find out about upcoming programs or to arrange a class field trip.

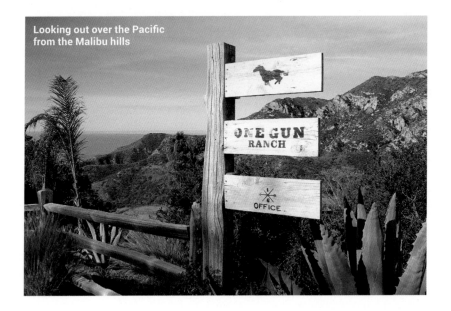
Looking out over the Pacific from the Malibu hills

37 **PRIMAL PASTURES**

42149 Elm St., Murrieta, CA 92562; 951-297-9933, primalpastures.com;
open year-round for prescheduled tours, workshops, and events.
Visit the website to see what's coming up.

WHAT THEY OFFER Classes and workshops, farm stand,
seasonal events, tours

WHAT HAPPENS WHEN A CLOSE-KNIT FAMILY with a can-do attitude
have a tough time finding pasture-raised chickens for sale? They start
their own farm, of course. Primal Pastures was born when Farmer Tom,
along with sons Jeff, Rob, and son-in-law Paul—practically on a whim—
starting raising 50 chicks on a leased parcel in Temecula. Because so
many other people in the community were searching for the same thing
(i.e., humanely raised meat), the operation grew exponentially. Today the
family raise hundreds of pastured meat and egg-laying chickens, along
with free-roaming herds of pigs, sheep, and cattle on 40 acres in Murrieta, as well as on several other properties throughout the state. They're
doing a heck of a job, too, especially considering they had zero farming
experience just a few years ago.

This family of farmers are clearly passionate about what they're doing,
and attribute their relatively quick success in large part to an unwavering
devotion to the principles upon which they founded the farm. Although
the farming practices at Primal Pastures are clearly biodynamic and
regenerative, the farmers aren't keen on using labels and prefer to think
of what they're doing as simply raising animals in their natural environment, the way it was done 100 years ago. And because they're so eager
to spread the gospel of farming the old-fashioned way, the brothers regularly open the farm for tours so that members of the community can see
firsthand what that looks like.

The tours are popular, drawing large groups of all ages, and fun—the
farm is loaded with cute, cuddly animals, and the brothers are, frankly,
pretty easy on the eyes themselves. They also have the natural rapport
that only siblings do, punctuating the tour with entertaining stories of the
trial and error that came with starting this whole endeavor. But the stars

of the show are probably the livestock guardian dogs, a family of regal Great Pyrenees–Anatolian Shepherd mixes that are as beautiful as they are friendly (although you can be assured that, should any predator come creeping around the livestock unannounced after dark, these watchdogs are quick to do their job). Visitors are first introduced to the baby chicks in the brooder, and then to the older chickens in custom-built chicken tractors on the pasture. The tractors are roomy, offering both shelter and fresh air for the birds, and are moved to a fresh patch of pasture every week, leaving the land fertilized with chicken manure for new growth, which the free-roaming pigs will eventually eat. It's a simple yet brilliant setup that leaves one wondering why factory farms have to exist at all.

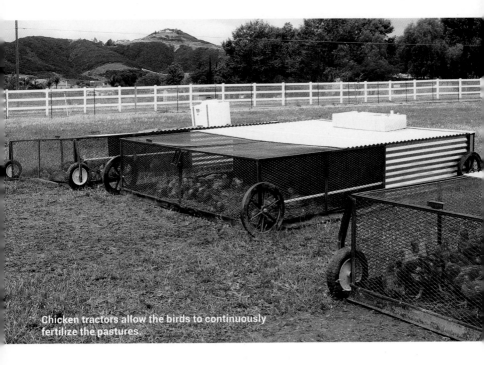

Chicken tractors allow the birds to continuously fertilize the pastures.

Primal Pastures specializes in heritage breeds, which are carefully selected for characteristics that will allow them to thrive in the subtropical climate of Riverside County, which is to say, extreme heat in the summer. The pigs are Kunekune, from New Zealand; the sheep are Dorper, from South Africa, and shed their coats naturally as opposed to needing shearing; and the milking cows are Jersey, which produce less volume but incredibly delicious, rich-tasting milk. Of course, there's no getting around the fact that, no matter how lovely of a life these animals have on the farm, they are—with the exception of the milking cows and laying hens—being raised to be eaten. The animals aren't processed on the premises, but the brothers are extremely discriminating about which USDA facilities they work with to ensure that the painstaking manner in which they raised their animals isn't rendered pointless by sloppy or inhumane slaughter practices. And for anyone who wants to have a deeper understanding of how our food moves from pasture to plate, Primal Pastures hosts semiregular chicken-processing workshops.

The farm tour typically lasts about an hour and a half and ends at the barn, where many of Primal Pastures products are available for purchase, including raw wildflower honey, eggs, sausages, chickens (whole and in parts), and just about any cut of beef or lamb you might desire, along with handmade bath and body products. The meat isn't cheap—nothing that's raised with this much care and attention is. But it is delicious; guaranteed you will taste the difference between these products and anything you'd buy at the grocery store. In fact, you will quite possibly be inspired to avoid conventionally raised meat altogether when you see how much greener the grass is (figuratively, of course, considering California's drought conditions) here at Primal Pastures.

NEARBY ATTRACTION Temecula Olive Oil Company

Temecula's wine country is just 15 minutes away from Murrieta. Although it can get busy on the weekends, Old Town Temecula is a charming and a convenient place to grab a bite and, if you're so inclined, do some wine tasting. While you're there, be sure to visit the Temecula Olive Oil tasting room, where you can sample a seemingly endless variety of olive oils and balsamic vinegars, direct from the growers. The tasting room servers are full of great recipe suggestions and eager to introduce clients to new flavors.

28653 Old Town Front St., Temecula, CA 92590; 951-693-4029, temeculaoliveoil.com

TIPS Bring a cooler or insulated bag if you think you might purchase meat at the end of the tour, especially if you're visiting in the warm season. Also, wear shoes or boots that you don't mind getting dirty, as you will be walking through chicken and pig poop when you tour the pastures.

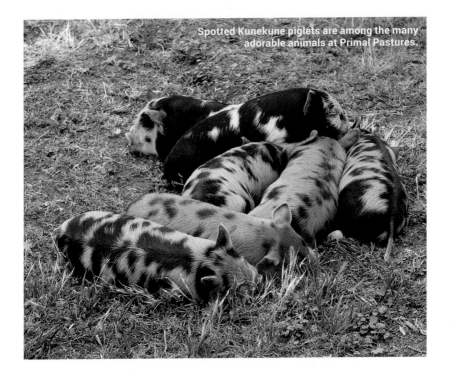

Spotted Kunekune piglets are among the many adorable animals at Primal Pastures.

38 SUZIE'S FARM

2570 Sunset Ave., San Diego, CA 92154; 619-662-1780, suziesfarm.com;
open year-round

WHAT THEY OFFER CSA, farm stand, tours, U-pick

LOCATED JUST ABOUT A MILE from the US–Mexico border and adjacent to the Tijuana River Valley Regional Park is Suzie's Farm, a modestly sized but efficient family-run operation that answers the San Diego area's call for sustainably and organically grown local produce. The farm was founded in 2004 by husband and wife Robin Taylor and Lucila De Alejandro, who named it after a dog they found on the property and then adopted. Robin and Lucila began their agricultural career with Sun Grown Organic, a sprout and wheatgrass operation that is still located across the road. Suzie's Farm has since grown to include 140 acres, several more farm dogs, and dozens of employees who grow herbs, fruits, and vegetables to be sold through their CSA, at their farm stand, and at farmers markets and a few local grocery stores. The farm is also open for U-pick and farm tours on Tuesday and Saturday.

While the landscape is certainly pastoral, Suzie's Farm doesn't concern itself with being pretty; fields are allowed to go fallow for two to three months at a time to rest the land between growing crops. The farmers consciously choose to fallow the fields rather than sow cover crops in order to save water; this is Southern California, after all. Because it's so frequently warm and sunny here, visitors are advised to wear hats and sunscreen and bring a bottle of water. A small eucalyptus grove near the parking area offers welcome relief from the sunshine, along with a hammock, tree swing, and tepee for kids to play in.

But the real action is on the one-hour farm tour, when kids and adults alike are educated about modern sustainable-farming practices and then encouraged to pick fresh produce to their hearts' content. Your guide will explain how the fields are managed and irrigated, introduce you to the flock of 500 pastured chickens, and share tricks of the organic farming trade, such as using ladybugs and essential oils of

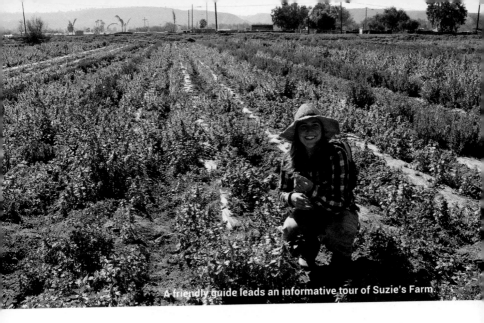

A friendly guide leads an informative tour of Suzie's Farm.

rosemary and peppermint for pest control and relying on birds of prey to manage the pesky gopher population. One of the interesting practices at Suzie's Farm is the permissive attitude toward plants that would be considered weeds on most conventional farms—you may be instructed on how to harvest and eat stinging nettle without getting stung, for example—and the emphasis on cultivating drought-tolerant native herbs such as lavender, rosemary, and thyme. Your tour is also likely to introduce you to vegetables that you might not have tried or even heard of before. The farm grows a diverse array of greens, each with its own distinctive flavor and texture, and you'll be encouraged to sample everything before harvesting as much as you can fill your bag with.

TIP In addition to weather-appropriate clothing and sun protection, visitors to Suzie's Farm must wear closed-toe shoes suitable for tramping through the dirt—no sandals or flip-flops are permitted on tours, no matter how hot it is. You might also consider bringing a picnic lunch to enjoy at one of the tables shaded by eucalyptus trees.

39 TANAKA FARMS

5380¾ University Drive, Irvine, CA 92612; 949-653-2100, tanakafarms.com; open spring, summer, and fall

WHAT THEY OFFER CSA, farm stand, kids' activities and attractions, seasonal events, tours, U-pick

TANAKA FARMS IS THE TYPE of agricultural endeavor that is sometimes referred to as "agritainment" and caters to families with young children by offering seasonal events with lots of value-added activities. That means you can pick strawberries in the spring, take a watermelon tour in the summer, visit a pumpkin patch in the fall, and select your Christmas tree in the winter. Tanaka closes for a brief period during winter before reopening in February with an open house to introduce the public to the coming year's programs and events.

The 30-acre farm is owned and operated by a third-generation Japanese American family and offers a rare glimpse of farm life in the heart of rapidly developing, suburban Orange County. Tanaka Farms made the switch to organic farming in 1998 when it changed locations in Irvine due to land development. Its produce is available through a CSA; subscribers can either pick up their weekly box at the farm or one of its pickup locations, or have it delivered directly to their home within the surrounding communities. Although the box may include fruits and vegetables from other growers besides the Tanaka family, it is all either certified organic or pesticide-free.

Visitors to Tanaka Farms will, however, find both organic and conventionally grown produce at the farm stand. In an effort to offer a broad selection of fruits and vegetables, Tanaka supplements its offerings with nonorganic items from other farms. Fortunately, everything is clearly labeled, so you can easily avoid produce of dubious provenance if you prefer to stick to certified organic, locally grown goods.

Tanaka Farms is undoubtedly a kid-friendly, one might even say kid-centric, destination. Families can tour the farm in a tractor-drawn wagon, find their way through a corn maze, or even ride pint-sized ATVs and John Deere Gators. Up front near the farm stand and gift shop, you'll find a petting zoo and carnival games. Be warned that all activities cost extra—during seasonal events, there is definitely a bit of a farm-meets-county-fair vibe. But you can also stick to a simple guided U-pick tour, during which the tractor will pull you around on a wagon for free, and you simply pay for the produce you pick, gaining an education in farming along the way.

Tanaka Farms is one of only a few places in the Los Angeles–Orange County area that give people the opportunity to actually pick pumpkins from the vine—a pleasurable novelty for most suburbanites and urban dwellers, who usually don't have any choice but to pick up their Halloween gourds at the supermarket.

TIP When shopping at the farm stand, pay attention to the posted signs and stick to buying the produce that was grown organically right there at Tanaka Farms.

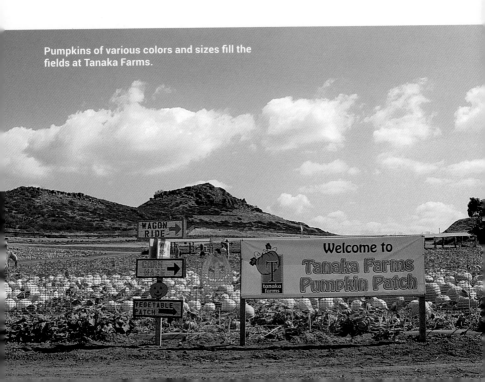

Pumpkins of various colors and sizes fill the fields at Tanaka Farms.

UNDERWOOD FAMILY FARMS

3370 Sunset Valley Road, Moorpark, CA 93021, 805-529-3690;
5696 Los Angeles Ave., Somis, CA 93066; 805-386-4660,
underwoodfamilyfarms.com; open spring, summer, and fall

WHAT THEY OFFER Camps, CSA, farm stand, kids' activities and attractions, special events, tours, U-pick

FOR MANY LOS ANGELES KIDS, UNDERWOOD FARMS is their first taste of farming life. This highly regarded, family-owned operation has been in the agritourism/agritainment game for a long time now, and holds a place on many parents' spring and summer break to-do lists. Like many farms targeted toward children, Underwood pulls out all the stops and draws huge crowds to seasonal events such as the Fall Harvest Festival and Christmas and Easter celebrations. But the farm educates and entertains the public throughout most of the year, as well, with school tours, day camps, U-pick fruit and vegetable fields, and even a farm animal show. This is also a highly productive working farm that supplies its produce to farmers markets all over Los Angeles and Ventura Counties and offers a CSA program with multiple pickup locations.

Underwood has two farms located about 10 miles apart and just under an hour northeast of Los Angeles. Moorpark is home to the Animal Center and most of the tyke-targeted rides and entertainment. For a modest admission fee, kids can climb on hay pyramids, grassy hills, play structures, and a combine harvester slide and enjoy the spectacle of a menagerie of farm animals, including donkeys, sheep, goats, chickens, ducks, birds, rabbits, cows, pigs, horses, emus, and alpacas. The goats, in particular, are a hoot to watch as they cross overhead on the elevated planks and ramps of their enclosure. Admission is a little higher on weekends and during holidays but also includes a tractor-drawn wagon ride around the farm and an animal show. For an additional fee, kids can also enjoy pony rides, electric train and tractor rides, a tricycle track, and a bouncy house. But Underwood isn't just for kids. The farm grows an impressively diverse array of fruits and vegetables throughout the year, much of it available to U-pick customers. A complete pick-your-own crop calendar is available on the website.

Meanwhile, the original location in Somis—open since 1980—specializes in U-pick blueberries. The Somis farm also has its own modest animal center, home to donkeys, alpacas, rabbits, and pygmy goats, and doesn't charge admission (although customers do, of course, pay for what they pick).

Neither of Underwood's farms is certified organic, although the company proudly claims to adhere to sustainable farming methods. This includes composting, cover cropping, and what is called "integrated pest management" (IPM), a practice that involves introducing beneficial insects and employing the use of the least-toxic insecticides, and only when absolutely necessary. More details about Underwood Family Farms' sustainable farming practices are available on its website.

Education and community involvement are guiding principles at Underwood. Most events and tours take place at the Moorpark location, including farm tours for school groups and summer farm camp for kids ages 4–10. Both locations also have a year-round farm stand selling fresh produce, pickles, eggs, nuts, and honey to locals and visitors alike.

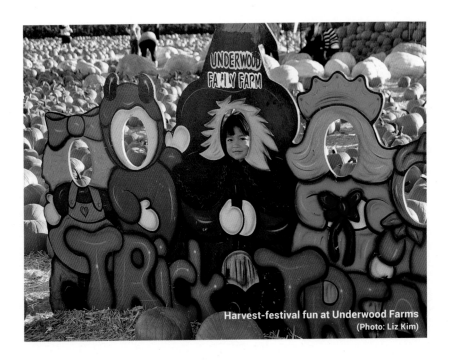

Harvest-festival fun at Underwood Farms
(Photo: Liz Kim)

41 WILD WILLOW FARM

2550 Sunset Ave., San Diego, CA 92154; sandiegoroots.org (no phone);
open year-round; detailed driving directions: tinyurl.com/wildwillowfarm

WHAT THEY OFFER Classes and workshops, CSA, tours, training and
internships, volunteer opportunities

JUST ACROSS THE STREET and down a short dirt road from Suzie's
Farm (see page 140) is Wild Willow Farm, a community farm and education center operated by a nonprofit called the San Diego Roots Sustainable Food Project. True to its name, Wild Willow is designed to exist
in harmony with the surrounding nature preserve in the Tijuana River
estuary, and the 6-acre farm has the feel of a thriving community garden that is a constant and beautiful work in progress. Visit Wild Willow
on a Saturday anytime of the year and you may see volunteers pulling
weeds, farm school attendees learning about compost, kids painting
rocks in the children's garden, or teenagers tending to goats. This bustling sense of community is what you get when you create a place that
is dedicated to educating the public about sustainable agriculture.

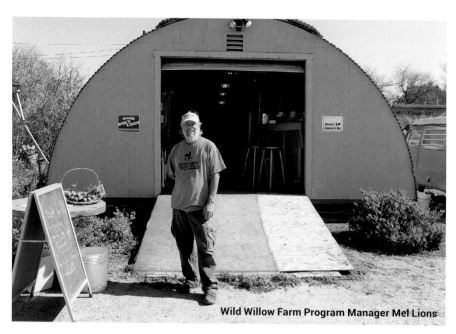

Wild Willow Farm Program Manager Mel Lions

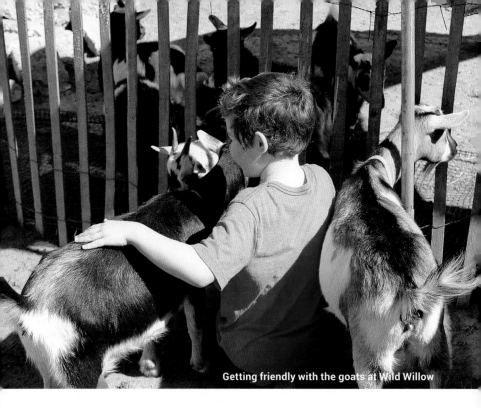
Getting friendly with the goats at Wild Willow

Much like at Suzie's, Wild Willow relies on natural selection to control pesky crop-eating critters, and you'll see raptor perches and owl and bat boxes erected around the premises. A fire pit is surrounded by cob benches, which will eventually break back down into the natural environment when they are no longer needed. A small herd of goats live on the farm, a couple of which are milked by hand once a day. Their milk is then used to make cheese and for soap-making workshops.

In keeping with its commitment to education, San Diego Roots runs the year-round Wild Willow School for Sustainable Farming. The program begins with a five-week Introduction to Farming course offered in partnership with the University of San Diego, which covers the fundamentals of sustainable farming and permaculture such as soil fertility, till and no-till strategies, composting, sowing and transplanting, irrigation, and pest control. After completing the intro, students can go on to enroll in more advanced courses, eventually culminating in the Farm Incubator program, which allows newbie farmers to use a portion of Wild Willow's land and take advantage of their direct marketing system to get a propitious start on running their own agricultural operations.

Of course, you don't need to commit to farm school to visit Wild Willow Farm. The farm hosts open volunteer days every Saturday, and the mood is open, friendly, and welcoming. Volunteers of all ages are welcome (although children should be supervised) and get to dig right in, so to speak—the day may involve weeding, mulching, composting, planting or feeding the goats or chickens. Volunteer coordinators provide gloves and any tools you may need, along with guidance and instruction. Volunteers are advised to wear closed-toe shoes and sun hats and to bring their own water bottles to fill up at the farm. Depending on the day, a potluck lunch may even be served with fresh-baked bread from the outdoor brick oven. Wild Willow also hosts regular community potluck dinners spring—fall.

If you'd rather visit the farm without supplying any labor and you can pull together a group of 10 people or more, then schedule a private farm tour. Tours cost a nominal fee per person and can be customized to suit the group's interests and curiosity. Large group tours of Wild Willow Farm are also offered, as are school field trips.

ADDITIONAL FARMS IN THE AREA

Coastal Roots Farm

441 Saxony Road, Encinitas, CA 92024; 760-479-6505,
coastalrootsfarm.org

The Leichtag Foundation headquarters is situated on nearly 70 acres of prime agricultural-zoned property in the lovely seaside town of Encinitas. A highly collaborative Jewish nonprofit organization dedicated to advancing social justice and a welcoming attitude toward interfaith families, Leichtag is uniquely positioned to advance self-sufficiency and agricultural innovation in San Diego County. To that end, the foundation incubates the Coastal Roots Farm nonprofit on the property. At the time of publication, the farm was still in the process of growing and expanding its offerings. Recurring events already include free twice-monthly tours of the ranch and monthly "Farm and Hang Out" events open to the public, as well as agricultural workshops grounded in progressive Jewish values. Some of the programs and building plans in store include day camps for kids; volunteering, internship, and apprenticeship opportunities; an outdoor kitchen and classroom; goat and sheep pens and milking parlors; a children's nature play area; and an 8-acre food forest to serve the surrounding community. Visit the website to see what programs and opportunities are currently offered.

Coral Tree Farm

598 Park Lane, Encinitas, CA 92024; 951-445-2342, coraltreefarm.com

This small suburban farm and nursery produces heirloom vegetables and tropical fruits in the pleasant coastal climate of San Diego County. Coral Tree also raises heritage breed goats and pastured chickens. The farm is open to the community twice a week and offers a farm-share program for locals interested in regularly receiving its organically and locally grown fruits, vegetables, and eggs.

Da-Le Ranch

24895 Baxter Ranch Road, Lake Elsinore, CA 92532; 951-657-3056, da-le-ranch.com

This sustainable family farm in the Inland Empire raises pastured, grass-fed beef and lamb, along with pigs, rabbits, chickens, and other fowl. They take a passionate stance against feedlots and contained area farming operations (CAFOs) and, to that end, have expanded from a single residential working farm to a small but multiple-location operation that continues to grow. Da-Le's meats can be purchased at area farmers markets or through a CSA package. Farm tours are available by appointment. Visit the website to find out when the next tour is offered and to sign up.

Friend's Ranch

15150 Maricopa Highway, Ojai, CA 93023; 805-646-2871, friendsranches.com

The Friend family has been growing citrus in the Ojai Valley for five (going on six) generations, offering a diverse selection of produce, including oranges, tangerines, mandarins, tangelos, lemons, grapefruit, and avocados. The packing house and store, where you can purchase fruit, honey, and other locally grown goodies, is open every Tuesday and Friday morning, and tours of the orchards are available starting in the spring.

Julian's Apple Orchards

Visit julianca.com for a calendar of upcoming events and list of attractions.

Much like Oak Glen in the Inland Empire and Apple Hill in the Sacramento area, Julian is the go-to autumn apple-picking spot for San Diego County. This old gold-mining town in the Cuyamaca Mountains about an hour east of San Diego is home to several orchards, such as Peacefield, Apple Starr, and Calico Ranch, that are open seasonally for apple picking, cider, and pie, and features year-round attractions such as gold mining, wine tasting, hiking, boating, and fishing.

Lombardi Ranch

29527 Bouquet Canyon Road, Saugus, CA; 661-296-8697, lombardiranch.com

Lombardi Ranch's location—off the beaten path, yet conveniently accessible from the suburban subdivisions of the Santa Clarita Valley—makes it a popular seasonal destination for families. The main draw here is the harvest festival, which takes place every fall and features a pumpkin patch, hay bales for climbing, wagon rides, an impressive corn maze, bake sales, and more seasonal fun.

McGrath Family Farm

1012 W. Ventura Blvd., Camarillo, CA 93010; 805-983-0333, mcgrathfamilyfarm.com

Featuring a roadside produce stand, a CSA, and seasonal U-pick for strawberries, tomatoes, squash, and pumpkins, McGrath Family Farm has been farming on the Oxnard Plain and serving the community for four generations. In addition to farm tours for both private groups and schools, McGrath hosts regular hands-on farm education days to educate the public about all aspects of organic farming.

Pomona College Organic Farm

130 Amherst Ave., Claremont, CA 91711; 909-607-8341, farm.pomona.edu

Pomona College, a member of the esteemed Claremont Colleges Consortium, features an on-campus farm to give students hands-on experience with organic agriculture. The farm is open to visitors on weekday afternoons and offers free workshops, tours, and volunteer opportunities—all open and available to the public. Students also run a biweekly farm stand on campus, selling produce from the farm at low prices.

Sarvodaya Farms

1196 S. San Antonio Ave., Pomona, CA 91766; 909-660-3514, sarvodayafarms.com

This small urban demonstration farm in Pomona is dedicated to educating the community about regenerative farming, offering a farmer-training program as well as volunteer opportunities and free community workshops. Sarvodaya's produce can be purchased through its CSA program.

Tapia Bros. Farm Stand

5251 Hayvenhurst Ave., Encino, CA 91436; 818-905-6155 (no website)

This family-owned and -operated farm and produce stand is right next to US 101 at the intersection of Hayvenhurst and Burbank, making it an incredibly convenient stop for San Fernando Valley dwellers, travelers, and commuters alike to pick up fresh produce. The farm offers seasonal attractions throughout the year, including a pumpkin patch, Christmas tree sales, and the popular Tomatomania festival. Call ahead to find out what's happening, as the produce stand is open only seasonally.

Urban Homestead

631 Cypress Ave., Pasadena, CA 91103; 626-795-8400,
urbanhomestead.com

The Dervaes family runs Urban Homestead out of their modest-size Craftsman home in suburban Pasadena. They claim to produce three tons of organic produce per year from their 0.1-acre garden, available for purchase at their front porch farm stand, and offer workshops on subjects like raising chickens, making bone broth, and brewing kombucha. The Dervaeses even host monthly "hootenannies" for the community. The events are a throwback to another time, right down to the pioneer-era garb donned by some of the family members.

Villa del Sol

6989 Elizabeth Lake Road, Leona Valley, CA 93551; 661-270-1356,
upickcherries.com

This 25-acre cherry orchard between Santa Clarita and Lancaster offers several varieties of sweet cherries for picking, including Bing, Rainier, Brooks, and Tulare, and sells its own raw honey. The orchard usually opens to the public for U-pick in May, but call ahead or check the website to make sure the fruit is ready to be harvested.

A BRIEF GLOSSARY OF SUSTAINABLE-FARMING TERMINOLOGY

ANIMAL WELFARE APPROVED (AWA) This certification and label for farms and their meat and dairy products ensures that "the animals were raised to meet the highest animal welfare and environmental standards" (as defined on animalwelfareapproved.org). AWA standards include high-welfare slaughter practices and pasture access for all animals, and certified farms are audited to ensure that they are following all required practices.

BIODYNAMIC AGRICULTURE This organic farming method developed by Dr. Rudolf Steiner in the 1920s is based on nurturing a relationship between the soil, plants, and animals to create a fully diversified, integrated, self-nourishing system. Key practices of this method include creating very specific homeopathic herbal and mineral preparations that are added to the compost, and determining the planting schedule according to the astrological calendar.

CERTIFIED ORGANIC Organic certification is awarded by the USDA to growers who meet a specific set of predefined agricultural standards. Requirements for this certification include absolutely no use of synthetic fertilizers and pesticides in the case of plants, and 100% organic feed and no administered antibiotics and hormones in the case of animals. Certified-organic foods must also be free of any genetically modified organisms (GMOs), which means genetically modified seed cannot be used.

COVER CROPPING Cover crops are legumes, grains, and grasses that are planted in between cash crops to serve several purposes, including suppressing weed growth, decreasing runoff, nitrogen fixing, and breaking up hard, dry soil. Common cover crops include buckwheat, rye, oats, hairy vetch, and red clover.

GRASS-FED/GRASS-FINISHED Conventionally raised cattle are typically fed a diet of corn and other grains, usually in a feedlot as opposed to outdoors in a natural environment. Grass-fed animals are allowed to graze outdoors—also known as foraging—on pasture, and may also be fed alfalfa hay when they are kept indoors during cold or inclement weather. Beef labeled "grass-fed" may have received a supplemental diet of grain prior to slaughter, whereas beef labeled "grass-finished" ate an exclusive diet of forage.

PASTURED/PASTURE-RAISED This description indicates that the animals were raised in an outdoor environment and got their nutrition from natural sources like grass and (in the case of omnivores, such as chickens) bugs, although some pasture-raised animals receive supplemental feed, particularly during the winter months. Animals often have access to shelter at night or during inclement weather. Pastured livestock differ from those labeled "free-range" or "cage-free" in that they live and feed primarily outdoors, as opposed to simply having access to the outdoors, which they may or may not actually use.

POLYCULTURE This agricultural practice emulates natural ecosystems by growing several types of crops in the same area. Common strategies include companion-planting fruits and vegetables that benefit one another and including beneficial weeds among the other crops.

ROTATIONAL GRAZING This process of moving livestock from one pasture to another prevents the land from being overgrazed and allows the vegetation to regenerate so that the land isn't depleted.

SUSTAINABLE/REGENERATIVE AGRICULTURE *Sustainable* is a broad farming term that usually indicates that food is grown and raised in a way that doesn't deplete the natural resources of soil and water. Practices often include composting, cover cropping, rotational grazing, drip irrigation, the use of beneficial insects and animals to control pests, and the avoidance of chemical fertilizers, herbicides, and pesticides. Regenerative agriculture takes things even further by actively building soil health to make the land even more fertile. Regenerative agriculture is often synonymous with "carbon farming," which is the attempt to sequester more carbon dioxide in the soil (and out of the atmosphere) by building more humus, or organic matter, into the soil.

INDEX

ABOUT THE AUTHOR

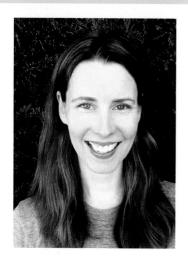

ERIN MAHONEY HARRIS is a mother, writer, and aspiring homesteader living in Santa Monica. She recently completed the UC Master Gardener training program and maintains an urban "microfarm" at home, growing an edible garden in an assortment of beds and containers and keeping quail for eggs. She and the kids would love to get a milking goat, but the neighbors aren't too keen on the idea. Ditto for beekeeping, although she hasn't given up on that dream just yet.

Erin has written about travel, urban farming, outdoor adventure, and sustainable living for *LA Parent* magazine, *The Huffington Post*, KCET.org, RedTri.com, and WeekendSherpa.com. She is currently working on the third edition of her popular guidebook *Walking L.A.: 38 Walks Exploring Stairways, Streets, and Buildings You Never Knew Existed* (Wilderness Press).

Follow @VisitCaliFarms on Twitter to keep up with Erin's farm visits and agritourism news, and check visitcalifarms.com for the latest updates on the farms featured in this book.